Serial Killers

The True Stories of Serial Killers and Why They Did It

(Exploring the Horrific Crimes of Little Known Murderers)

Carolyn Collins

Published By **Bella Frost**

Carolyn Collins

All Rights Reserved

Serial Killers: The True Stories of Serial Killers and Why They Did It (Exploring the Horrific Crimes of Little Known Murderers)

ISBN 978-1-77485-528-7

No part of this guidebook shall be reproduced in any form without permission in writing from the publisher except in the case of brief quotations embodied in critical articles or reviews.

Legal & Disclaimer

The information contained in this ebook is not designed to replace or take the place of any form of medicine or professional medical advice. The information in this ebook has been provided for educational & entertainment purposes only.

The information contained in this book has been compiled from sources deemed reliable, and it is accurate to the best of the Author's knowledge; however, the Author cannot guarantee its accuracy and validity and cannot be held liable for any errors or omissions. Changes are periodically made to this book. You must consult your doctor or get professional medical advice before using any of the suggested remedies, techniques, or information in this book.

Upon using the information contained in this book, you agree to hold harmless the Author from and against any damages, costs, and expenses, including any legal fees potentially resulting from the application of any of the information provided by this guide. This disclaimer applies to any damages or injury caused by the use and application, whether directly or indirectly, of any advice or information presented, whether for breach of contract, tort, negligence, personal injury, criminal intent, or under any other cause of action.

You agree to accept all risks of using the information presented inside this book. You need to consult a professional medical practitioner in order to ensure you are both able and healthy enough to participate in this program.

Table of Contents

Chapter 1: Long Island Serial Killer 1

Chapter 2: The Redhead Murderer 25

Chapter 3: Alphabet Murders 40

Chapter 4: Highway Of Tears............................. 60

Chapter 5: Freeway Phantom 82

Chapter 6: Alabama: Sherry Lynn Marler 100

Chapter 7: Colorado: Pageant Queen Jonbenet Ramsey... 114

Chapter 8: Connecticut: Mary Badaracco Disappeared 139

Chapter 9: Delaware: Jane Marie Prichard 155

Chapter 10: Georgia: Vanessa "Honey" Malone 170

Chapter 11: Hawaii: Lisa Au's Murder 178

Conclusion 183

Chapter 1: Long Island Serial Killer

Alias Craigslist Strangler

Locality: Long Island, NY

Time-frame: 1996 to 2010 and possibly to 2013.

Victims: 10 - 16

being isolated from the bustling and internationally recognized New York city by the Long Island Sound, one might think Long Island to be a peaceful and tranquil alternative to the city that is never asleep. However, the region remains a very populated island that is location of two of the three main airports in those in the New York Metropolitan area: LaGuardia and JFK International Airport.

A vast landmass that is which is surrounded by water offers the benefits of beaches. Ah beaches… the perfect location for families to enjoy an enjoyable day or for people to enjoy an entire day in the sunshine. Long Island beaches are renowned for their white sand, fineness beaches, rails for the beach, breathtaking waves at the ocean, public places for picnics, and visually beautiful sunsets and sunrises.

But, the Long Island residents Long Island were hit by waves of shock and terror at the time that one of their beaches on which they were able to find peace and joy was used as the backdrop for one of a sequences of the most sinister incidents to ever occur within the United States of America.

What can turn an incredible place like Long Island into a nightmare for the residents of Long Island?

What were those who suffered from this homicidal madman?

Murders

Authorities in Suffolk found 10 bodies at Gilgo beach There had been a variety of theories about being the Long Island serial killer being responsible for additional deaths. For a better comprehension of Gilgo beach tragedy we will look at the incident that triggered the investigation as well as those four people who were victims in those Long Island murders that were initially discovered close to Gilgo Beach.

Shanna Gilbert

Age 25 years old

A person who had a turbulent childhood Shanna Gilbert was born on 24th day of October in 1986, was youngest from four girls.

After moving to live together with her husband in the year 2007 Shanna was soon a part of an escort agency , while pursuing the desire to be an actor and a singer.

Shanna's time as an escort was not what could be described as smooth. In the course of three years Shanna experienced at least one arrest and was required to have an implant of titanium within her jaw after an incident during work. There are reports that claim Shanna was a drug addict in her time serving as an escort.

Craigslist was cited as the platform of choice to advertise their services for escorting. Shanna was believed to be charging $200 per hour, and according reports, she earned up to 600 dollars per night.

Shanna was employed as a driver by Joseph Brewer through craigslist on the 1st of May 2010, that led her to go to the residence of Joseph along alongside Michael Pak, who was a driver Shanna was working with.

There was a report about Shanna dialing 911 using a mobile phone in Joseph Brewer's house, where she also reached out to Michael Pak for help. Michael Pak who had driven Shanna to the Brewer residence and then stayed in the car throughout her visit was reported to have believed that Shanna was intoxicated and just stayed there.

But, to his surprise, after a time, he saw Shanna fled from Joseph Brewer's home and began banging on the doors of the neighbors of Joseph's. Michael was trying to track Shanna with his car however, Shanna was gone before she could be seen.

The neighbor who lived with Joseph Brewer said that he'd tried to dial 911, but Shanna would not allow him to make the call.

A few weeks after her violent outburst at the residence of Joseph Brewer and to the annoyance of her family members and officers, no sign of Shanna. The police were unable connect Joseph Brewer or Michael Pak to her disappearance because of the lack of evidence.

The horror slowly began to be spewed out through bone fragments of Long Island residence, when an investigator who was from Suffolk County while conducting a training session with the cadaver dog in Gilgo Beach, came across the remains of a deceased body on an area that was near to the residence of Joseph Brewer. What could Joseph Brewer have buried Shanna in his area?

The remains discovered did not have a titanium jawlike the one that Shanna did, proving they weren't Shanna's. There is no evidence linking Joseph Brewer to the disappearance of Shanna Gilbert.

The police following discovering the body started an exhaustive examination of the area. They received a shocking sight that could make the most shivering of hearts feel a sense of horror. Over the course of a few days, three additional bones were discovered close to 50 yards of each other. These bones were discovered wrapped in burlap bags.

On the 11th day of December 2011, one year following her disappearance, Shanna's remains were found about a half mile from the residence of Joseph Brewer in the area where she last saw her.

Amber Lynn Costello

Age 27 years old

The birthplace of Amber Lynn Overstreet In Charlotte born in Charlotte and born within Wilmington, North Carolina, Amber was a divorcee twice who was moved in to New York by her sister in the year 2019 as she battled with addiction to drugs.

The sister Katherine Overstreet explained that Amber was admitted to an sober home before she moved into her own apartment situated in North Babylon, New York.

Amber was reported as sexually active when she was just 17 years old. Katherine said that prostitution led her sister into darkness of addiction to drugs. This led to the fact that Amber continued to provide sexual services to get her next fix.

At the time she disappeared, Amber Lynn had received an email and bargained for $1,500 in sexual sex with the person. It was an amount that was higher than normal for this kind of job. Perhaps, being able to pay such an amount of money for the smallest task and quick fix has affected her judgement or perhaps she was simply reckless The phone call caused her to abandon her caution and leave for the night.

It was revealed that Amber was using her roommate's phone to arrange a meeting to meet her client. Dave Schaller who had been Amber's roommate told the story that the client had contacted him around three or four times, which enticed Amber into the illusion of safety with the caller.

Amber was known to her roommate who had advertised her service on backpage.com as Southern belle. Dave told her that if the event was scheduled in a house or hotel then he would drive Amber to the location and leave the vehicle outside. In some instances, Dave would be allowed at the home of the client, and would be able to wait in the next room in the event that Amber require him. According to Dave at least one occasion, the clients threatened to commit violence, and Dave had to intervene.

Amber scheduled a meeting for her custodian on 2nd of September hoping to make some money fast. However, she was never able to make her way back home.

If Dave reached Amber's younger sister Katherine from North Caroline on the 3rd of September to inquire about Amber's location, Katherine told her she thought Amber was in a rehab facility and that her sister was not in contact for the duration of her rehabilitation.

Amber Costello was identified as one of the four bodies that were discovered at the bottom of Gilgo Beach in December 2010.

Melissa Barthelemy

Age 24-year-old

Growing up from Upstate New York, Melissa was a graduate at South Park High School, Buffalo as well as the cosmetology license which was a short time ago able her to earn a living at Supercuts. Melissa was believed to have dreamed of running her own salon. At the age of twenty, Melissa moved to the Bronx in 2007.

Since the time she was born, Melissa worked as an escort, posting her services for sale on Craigslist. Melissa's uncle told her that Melissa was a fan of New York City and had an affinity for shopping, in which he described her as "a person who shops."

In the evening of the 10th July, the 10th of July in 2010, Melissa had scheduled the meeting with a client who had made a deposit of $900 into her account at the bank. The report said that Melissa attempted to call her former boyfriend however, the was never answered.

Melissa did not make it home that night.

After Melissa's disappearance, she and her teenage daughter, Amanda, began receiving unwanted calls from a mysterious person calling her and taunting Amanda with words such as "Melissa is dead , and I'm going observe her decay."

The authorities tracked these calls and located Madison Square Garden and Massapequa However, who was the person who made the calls was not determined.

Maureen Brainard-Barnes

Age 25 years old

Maureen Brainard-Barnes was born at Groton, Connecticut. She was a divorced mom of two children aged age eight and one in the year that she vanished. Her sister said that Maureen has been a prolific reader who was prone to poetry and lyricism as got older.

Maureen was viewed as a very loving and caring person by her sibling. Maureen was employed as a seller at Foxwoods Resort Casino where she then quit and began caring for her first child, while her husband was working.

When Maureen was pregnant with two children, the mother was working as a cashier and telephone marketer as well as developing her model portfolio. Just before she disappeared, Maureen had been fired from her last job as an telemarketer. Not able to find a replacement job and in arrears with her monthly rent payments Maureen was forced to take on sex jobs in order to live.

Maureen Like the other victims, lived within Norwich, Connecticut. But, she was last found in the Super 8 Hotel Manhattan on the 9th July 2007, in which she was staying for the night. Maureen was at the hotel in order to schedule her first meeting with the client she found on Craigslist. According to the reports, Maureen was supposed to return to Norwich the following day, but she did not make it.

Megan Waterman

Age Age: 22 years old

Megan Waterman, who had been born at Scarborough Maine, much like Maureen Brainard Barnes, who was not an habitant in New York. There was a report that Megan along with her partner Akeem Cruz had made the trip in New York over the Memorial Day weekend. She was last seen in the Hotel situated in Hauppauge, Long Island.

Megan's mom had said that it wasn't the first time that her daughter had been to New York with her boyfriend and Megan was aware of the dangers of having her information as an escort publicized on the internet.

The police reports indicated that Megan was being snatched to have sex by her boyfriend.

In the course of investigating this investigation, Detective Blatchford was concerned that Megan's Craigslist advertisements could be the cause of her disappearance.

Megan was reported missing on June 6, 2010 and it was revealed that she had texted her boyfriend of 20 years that she was headed out and that she would call him later that morning. Six months later, after her disappearance, the body of Megan was discovered on Gilgo beach along with the other victims. The reason for her death was found to be strangulation.

Modus Operandi

The majority of victims of Long Island serial killer shared the physical characteristics of an Caucasian woman, and were involved in the sexual trade. The bodies of the victims were found to be strangled by perhaps an unidentified black belt which was left at the scene of the crime.

In every rule, there are exceptions. For instance, in the case of Long Island serial killer, this would be the demise of an unidentified young Asian man, who had been dressed in feminine clothes. The victim was thought to be a prostitute, and the reason for his death was trauma from blunt force. Additionally, there was an infant girl who was believed to range between

16-24 months. Her death was caused by unproven causes. DNA tests confirmed that she was the child of the victim.

In the past, Long Island serial killer used "burlap bags" to eliminate his victims, many of whom were later dismembered. The perpetrator chose his preferred location of the Ocean Parkway near Gilgo Beach in Suffolk County as his destination to dump his victims.

There is a strong indication that The Long Island serial killer as an organised criminal who made plans and then executed the murders. The killer would reach out to his victims via Craigslist and then meet them on his terms, kill themand then take their remains to the destination of choice to dispose of them.

The analysis of the behavior for The Long Island serial killer revealed that he was an Caucasian person in their 30s or 40s. Based on this the fact that it was likely that the perpetrator was educated and knowledgeable about computers. According to the evidence that the perpetrator would be extremely familiar with the geographical features and geography of Long Island.

After getting caught, after stalking Melissa Barthelemy's sister using the victim's cellphone, police traced the phone calls to midtown Manhattan and been a source of suspicion that the perpetrator may be in Manhattan.

This Long Island serial killer has been speculated to have similar behaviors with Ted Bundy. This type of killer is considered to be extremely sexual Psychopaths with a love for killing that is so strong that they can't stop.

Investigation

After discovering what was thought to be a horrifying discovery in the year the year 2001, authorities from Suffolk County, Long Island continued to search for more victims and found further remains of victims that seemed to be an endless nightmare.

When the fourth victim was discovered that was an infant believed to be between the age of 16-24 months, Nassau County and New York state police departments were required to participate in an investigation of the Long Island serial killings. The child was thought of as "Baby Doe".

Doe was a baby. Doe was found wrapped in the blanket. The police report stated that there were no visible evidence of trauma. Even though it didn't fit to the Modus Operations for The Long Island killer, the police could not eliminate the possibility of Baby Doe's death as a murder.

DNA tests were conducted to determine the identity of disembodied victims, while new remains continued to emerge as part of the investigation. On April 11, 2011, a dog of the police found the remains of a victim, identified as "Jane Doe number. 3" and included bones as well as a separate skull believed to be from another victim. The DNA test proved the Baby Doe's DNA was closely related to Jane Doe No. 3.

There was speculation in the police department that the murderer could be someone who had knowledge of police techniques came to light after the killer started following an individual's sister. The killer would call at brief intervals.

On December 10, 2015 The Suffolk County Police Department announced that the FBI was officially a part of the investigation after many years of non-official support to police.

The trails in investigation of the Long Island serial killer investigation are long-running cold. The authorities might have more information than they've been providing for the general public.

Suspects

In the course of the investigation into the killings that occurred in Long Island, several individuals appeared to be in the same mold of the perpetrator. But, with no concrete evidence there was no action taken or is being taken against the suspects. It should come as an unsurprising fact that while reading this article, you may have discovered suspicions from your personal experience. Are there others who share the same suspicions as you do? Let's discover. Here are a few suspects in the Long Island Killings.

Joseph Brewer

Being caught in the middle of the storm, which formed the catalyst for the case, Joseph Brewer was immediately identified as a suspect in the investigation due to the fact that Brewer was the one who appointed Shanna Gilbert to act as her escort in the evening that she disappeared.

In interrogations, Joseph Brewer maintained that Shanna was acting out in a bizarre manner prior to leaving his home. While speculators labelled Joseph Brewer as a person of interest, his position as suspect in the case was cleared when he passed the polygraph test administered by authorities.

John Bittrolff

A murder conviction was revoked several years earlier John Bittrolff was an suspect in the in the year 2017.

John Bittrolf had been sentenced to 25 years' imprisonment for prior murder charges however he was not in prison during the time that it was discovered that the Long Island Serial Killer investigation was in progress.

John Bittrolff had a previous history of killing two sexual people in the years 1993 and 1994, and was believed to have killed another victim. It was only natural John was a possible suspected suspect for one in the Long Island killings. Additionally, putting John as a suspected suspect was that he resided in Manorville in the same time frame that the first victims were murdered by the Long Island serial killer were killed.

James Bisset

Based on the notion that the Long Island serial murderer was skilled at throwing away bodies of victims' remains in burlap bags, James Bisset was fingered out as a possible suspect due to his position as co-owner of the largest provider of burlap sacks in the Long Island region , which was dubbed "Long Island Nursey."

What makes the story concerning James Bisset even more suspicious is the fact that he committed suicide just hours following Shanna Gilbert's corpse was discovered. Due to his suicide, police did not launch a formal inquiry into James Bisset's role in any murder. But, James Bisset had remained an individual of interest to investigators in the form of armchair detectives.

Robert Durst

Robert Durst was the heir to the New York City real-estate magnate and was thought of being the serial murderer. When he was a kid Robert's mother leapt (or there is a belief that they say she fell) onto the top of the house situated in Scarsdale, New York.

Robert who was only 7 years old, was the witness of this tragic incident. He also was required to undergo psychotherapy.

Robert was believed to have been a domineering violent spouse and she tried to break free from their toxic relationship. At the time Robert's wife, Kathleen, suddenly disappeared and her husband did not declare her missing for 4 days. Furthermore, Robert's description regarding the moment he met his wife was not consistent which caused a significant problem for police.

One of Robert's close friends and admirers was Susan Berman who was known to have grew up with criminals thanks to her book. in 2000 Susan died in the family home of her California home, and the reason for her death consisted of a single shot on the neck. It was easy to think that her death was an act of gang violence, but sources later discovered the fact that Susan Berman had been in contact with police regarding her disappearance. Kathleen Durst.

In the year his friend was killed, Robert posed as a female who was mute and adopted the name of his childhood acquaintance named Dorothy Ciner. Robert known as Dorothy Ciner moved to a unclean residence in Texas. It was discovered that Robert could sometimes appear as a mute person and switch identities.

Transferring to Texas It appears that trouble would follow wherever Robert was. in September of 2001 just after his move from Texas with the pseudonym Dorothy Ciner, he was again caught up in a fresh controversy. The remains of Dorothy's elderly friend, Morris Black, were discovered floating on the shores of the region that is Galveston and the body of the victim was never found.

A subsequent investigation resulted in police discovering the trail of blood that led from the residence of Black to Dorothy's residence. In the course of the course of this investigation that

Robert's name was discovered and he was detained.

While the remnants of Morris Black were disposed of in the same manner as those of Long Island killings, the FBI eventually failed to link Robert to the murders. He was exonerated of murdering his neighbour.

In the final verdict, Robert was convicted for the murder of his close friendship partner Susan Berman in September 2021 that resulted in him being sentenced to life in the California Health Care Facility.

There's a long number of people suspected in the Long Island serial killer case and it could be a lengthy book to look into each one in depth.

Conspiracy Theories

A variety of conspiracy theories regarding various conspiracy theories surrounding Long Island serial killings have emerged, many of which targeted the police department with good reason. The police department has been repeatedly criticized for muddled up the matter because of corrupt practices within its department.

James Burke, who had been an ex-Suffolk County police chief, was one of the suspects in the Long Island serial killings. Burke was well-known for his brutality and previous history with prostitutes. There was speculation that Burke may have erred in handling the matter as he tried to protect the FBI from coming in. This incident caused a lot of questions regarding the former chief's motives.

Burke was referred to repeatedly in the past as the Long Island Serial Killer , or in certain cases, an accomplice that was trying to sabotage the investigation because of his close connection to "rich and powerful" Oak Beach individuals who were responsible for the murders.

There are speculations that the murderer may be an insider of the police department, who was able to evade justice due to his intimate information about the case similar to the TV show character "Dexter".

Impacts

The never-ending search for bodies found by the authorities have left no trace of shock that swept across the residents in Long Island and the entire nation. It wasn't surprising to discover an initial shock led to a sense of terror and anxiety, as the people were battling the idea of a mysterious killer within their vicinity.

In the aftermath, there was a furore following several years of failed investigations into the incident and one major reason for public fury was the alleged involvement and corruption in the past the police commissioner James Burke.

A long-standing history of drug abuse and frequenting sex workers violence along with manipulations of the situation by repeatedly refusing to cooperate with the FBI and the police chief had put the population in a state of panic and was considered by journalist Jesse Kornbluth, who called him a uncivil animal.'

More than a year has passed after the beginning of these horrifying Long Island serial killings, the case is not solved. The case has triggered feelings of dismay for the general public, who find it a bit frightening that someone can go on a murder streak and not risk being arrested by authorities.

Chapter 2: The Redhead Murderer

Alias: Bible Belt Strangler

The location: Interstates across America

Time Frame: 1978 to the beginning of 1992

Victims: 6 - 11 (estimated)

joining the ranks of a mystifying serial murders in America The Redhead Murderer was a gruesome case that created alarm bells in the hearts of many people during the 80s. It was a case that spanned several states, including Kentucky, Arkansas, Pennsylvania, Mississippi, West Virginia and Tennessee the victims were women who were killed and later disposed of along interstates by a fugitive.

After months of finding bodies in their interstates police agencies of the affected states held an informal meeting to discuss how the bone-chilling issue can be dealt with the best way.

The redhead murders more difficult is the reality that the majority of the victims were unable to be identified, or it were too slow in identifying. The reports further suggest that the root of this issue was due to the location at which the bodies were discovered would not be close to the houses of the victims.

Although some may question whether or the deaths were simply coincidences, the vast majority of people would agree that somebody was targeting and killing women with one characteristic such as red or reddish hair.

The most frequently asked question was and remains: who was able to make a location like an interstate an ideal location for murders? Who were the poor souls who were victims of his brutality?

Murders

Like the name suggests the Redhead Murderer earned his name due to the string of murders that were not solved by redheaded women across the US. Many victims were hitchhikers, and theories were also suggested to suggest they were prostitutes.

As a lot of murders occurred on interstates, the police struggled to determine if they were all one suspect.

Then the list of eleven definitive victims was compiled and spread across five states over eight months. Through the compilation, four redhead women who were victimized at the hands of Fort Worth, Texas and one from Ohio had been omitted from this list.

Jane Doe

Age: 35 to 45 years old

Location found: Wetzel County, West Virginia

Jane Doe, the name is not known, is considered to be the first victim believed to be the Redhead murderer. On February 13, 1983 the body naked of an unknown Caucasian woman was discovered along Route 250 close to Littleton within West Virginia's Wetzel County.

Investigators, after multiple attempts, failed to identify Jane Doe. The dominant theory was that she might be a prostitute from Pittsburgh.

Jane Doe had been found by an elderly couple who initially thought of her body that was lying in the snow, face down like a mannequin which was dumped by the owner. The conclusion was not too far-fetched because trash was frequently placed in the area without permission.

Jane Doe, like many others who were victims of the Redhead Murderer was more auburn-colored hair rather than red. Jane Doe stood at 5 6 feet tall and weighed around 135 pounds.

An autopsy performed on Jane Doe showed that she was dead for several days, however the reason of her death was not determined. The speculations among the investigators in the case suggested that she was killed by strangulation.

Lisa Jarvis Nichols

Age 28 years old

Location located: West Memphis, Arkansas

A year following Jane Doe's discovery Jane Doe, Lisa Nichols was discovered by a motorist on Interstate 40 in close proximity to West Memphis, Arkansas. The reason for her death was found to have been strangulation. Lisa had just one sweater on when she was found which was in line with the fashion of the victims who are discovered naked.

It was speculated that she may have been on a ride before being killed. An informant from the jailhouse, who was referred to as pimp in media reports claims to have resided with Lisa for a time while she was living in West Memphis and helped in the identification of Lisa's body.

Popular with the Nashville Police Department, Lisa was said to possess the second-longest record of prostitutes within Nashville in addition to Davidson

County, thus falling into the category of those who were branded as prostitutes.

In the Florida prison when the search the pimp claimed that he have seen Lisa riding in the tractor-trailer of a truck stop located outside of Shearerville on September 12, 1984. Lisa who was blonde strawberry-colored hair that was blonde roots is believed to have been different from the other victims who had hair with reddish hues.

Campbell County Victim One: Tina Marie McKenney Farmer

Age: 17-30 years old

Location discovered: Campbell County, Tennessee

Campbell County seemed to have been the victim of the stick when it came to The Redhead Murders as they had not just one, but two victims in their area which raised eyebrows.

Tina was discovered on Interstate 75 close to Jellico near Jellico East Tennessee on the 1st of January, 1985. The woman was dressed in a white velour shirt with blue pants. It was suggested by the investigators that Tina was in a state of death for two or three days prior to her being found.

An autopsy performed on her found that Tina was strangled using rope. However, unlike the others, Tina hadn't suffered sexual abuse. There was also evidence that Tina was about twelve weeks pregnant at the time she was shot dead and that she was due to give birth recently.

As compared to other victims Tina has distinct characteristics among them were freckles, eyes that were green as well as a few marks. A few of the marks included a healing burn injury in the left hand, as well as a two-inch mark that appeared to be a little bit across her forehead, and an injury across her hand. She also shared the similar colour of her hair: red as the others who were injured.

Tina was lost by the family one day after the thanksgiving celebration in 1985. Her identity was not known until the year 2018 after she was recognized by fingerprints.

Campbell County Victim Two

Age: 9 to 15 years old

Location located: Jellico

The possibility of being a potential victim to the Redhead murderer, and possibly the youngest to date an additional victim was discovered by a passing motorist on the Big Wheel Gap Road near Jellico in April 1985. in the same area that was Tina Marie McKenney Farmer.

The victim's skeleton fragment was the only remains. 32 bones were found at the site of the discovery. Investigators concluded that she aged between nine and fifteen at the date of her death. They also believed it is likely that she was deceased for at least up to four years prior to the discovery.

Because of the condition of her body the condition of her body made it impossible to establish her physical features or the reason for her death. The only identifiable feature was a few dental fillings. The remains of a pair of hiking shoes and some jewelry were found close to the place of her body.

Despite the limitations created by the incomplete skeleton, doctors eventually were able to create the reconstruction of the face of the deceased.

Modus Operandi

The murderer was recognized for picking victims who were near to their families. If this was due to random chance, isn't established. There were a few inconsistencies that left it difficult to establish a motive to these murders. maybe the perpetrator was an inexperienced or uncoordinated individual or a nefarious perpetractor.

A number of victims were sexually assaulted prior to their deaths, while others were not, making one think that the motive was entirely sexually motivated.

Investigation

The unpredictability of the investigation made it appear as if the killings of the redheads could be coincidental, However, some clues been discovered that helped in establishing the link between the deaths.

The most important leads pursued by investigators was the similarity in the physical characteristics and characteristics of victims. The majority of them were between 20-40 years of age. They were identified as prostitutes or hitchhikers and their bodies were often found in close proximity to major roads, with the reason of death determined to be strangulation.

Female victims' bodies were discovered separated by hundreds of miles and prompted investigations to be carried out by various agencies under whose authority the findings were made.

Due to the fact that only one victim was known at that time, it became difficult to move forward with the investigation since the family members of the victim were not advocating for justice after the case was in limbo for quite a while.

The Redhead Murders remained cold cases until the summer of 2017, at which point the FBI began to re-examine the evidence from the 1985 murder. The re-examination revealed that an identical fingerprint was discovered on a refrigerator, however it was later discovered to not be related to the incident.

In spite of this setback the FBI began investigating the case with renewed determination. The theory was that the murderer was a truck driver who was based in Knoxville, Tennessee who would draw victims into his vehicle to strangle them using his hands, before throwing their bodies on the roadside.

The FBI was also able to find an article on a blog about the disappearance of a red-haired woman from Indiana. The woman's red hair was thought to be a match with what was described as Jane Doe's victim of Campbell County. Further examination revealed a DNA match to the fingerprint which was found earlier. They confirmed her identity by her initials Tina Farmer.

Suspects

The inconsistencies of The Redhead Murders brought about hindrances for the authorities , who had a difficult time coming up with the list of suspects. But, two suspects came up in the investigations. Meet:

Thomas Lee Elkins

In fitting into "Truck driver" stories, Thomas Lee Elkins, who was a long-haul truck driver from Tennessee and was brought into custody for questioning regarding The Redhead Murders in 1986 after being arrested at Dyers County just 80 miles north of Memphis. Thomas was arrested for abducting a woman aged 20 who had managed to escape from his truck.

Although Thomas was ruled out as suspects of the Redhead Murders, he was charged with kidnapping as well as sexual assault.

Jerry Leon Johns

Jerry Johns, another long-haul truck driver from Cleveland, Tennessee, was thought to be a possible person of interest in Redhead Murder cases.

Jerry was detained in 1985, after he kidnapped and attempted to kill an innocent woman from Knoxville. It was reported that the Knoxville woman Linda Schake, had been strangled by Jerry who was using an item of cloth was ripped off Linda's blouse. John then went on to suffocate Linda and then dragged her into a storm drain and died beneath Interstate 40 near Watt Road. Linda was believed to have had hair that was red which would fit the description of the other victims.

Authorities have reported that the knot on the fabric Jerry used to tie the knot on Linda was very similar to the fabric found in the neck area of Campbell County Victim Two just two months prior.

Unfortunately for Jerry and fortunate for Linda she was able to survive. Linda's survival resulted in the quick detention for Jerry Johns. The suspect was interrogated regarding the series of murders across the country and the account for the police detective Larry Johnson of the Knox County police department. Jerry's third statement during interrogation was "serial murderer".

Jerry Johns was referred to as an "extremely clever" criminal with a deep knowledge of the criminal justice system and immediately made reference to his curiosity about the psychological aspects of serial killers.

There was no evidence that linked Jerry to or any other Redhead murders, Jerry was found guilty of attempted and aggravated the murder Linda Schake and was sentenced to 73 years of prison. John passed away in the year 2015 while serving the jail sentence.

In 2019, DNA evidence was conclusively linking Jerry Johns to the murder of Tina Marie McKenney Farmer in 1985. This was after a semen samples were found inside Tina's clothes and was then added to the Combined DNA Index System (CODIS) and confirmed as a match to Jerry Johns' DNA.

Impacts

The random nature of the case has led to many speculations, not only from the authorities, but also from the general public. One participant from an online forum wrote:

"Not just is the murderer not known, but a number of victims are still not identified. The murders are an even more intriguing mystery. Don't get me wrong... I love a good mystery. Most good mysteries include an ending to bring things to the close. This one isn't."

Based on the position of the bodies of the victims Many speculated that the killer was an experienced truck driver. Many also believed that if the perpetrator was a trucker maybe he'd quit or just changed his route or changed to a different trucking company that he worked for.

As with other serial killings the motive behind Redhead Murders is not known. Redhead Murders has left people in an uneasy state without any idea of the motives is behind the murders.

Chapter 3: Alphabet Murders

Alias: Double Initial Killer

Location: Rochester, New York

Time Frame 1971 from 1971 to 1973

Victims: 3

Rochester is regarded as the third-highest populated city within the State of New York, ranked after NYC and Buffalo. The city was named in honor of the Colonel Nathaniel Rochester, the city was founded in 1817 , following the American Revolution.

It is possible that New York is a state that New York has been a place of refuge for psychopaths as well as serial killers who have a bloodlust that is comparable to the evil. However, that's an inaccurate stereotype to associate the people with.

Somehow, bizarre people enjoy murders for fun during their spare time. In the town of Rochester will have its own experience of terror and fear as the serial murderer chose to choose the area for his horrific crimes.

Murders

In contrast to the previous two serial killers we have revealed this one, the Double Initial Serial Killer has only a few victims. Maybe he just quit or moved to a different location to carry on his murderous spree We will never find out.

What causes the blood-curling of the Alphabet Murders the victims' choice. In the case of Double Initial, Double Initial killer had decided that Rochester, New York would be the ideal location for his kidnap, to sexually assault , and kill children.

Carmen Colon

Age 10 years old

In the mid-afternoon of November 1971, the young Carmen Colon was reported to be out conducting on errands. She went to the pharmacy to purchase medications for the mother of her. When she was told that the prescription for her mother was not ready, the pharmacist told her that Carmen was getting agitated and advised her to leave.

The pharmacist was thought to be the only person to talk to 10-year-old Carmen. The pharmacist also said that Carmen was a passenger in the back of a Ford Pinto that seemed to be waiting for her as she left the pharmacy.

The incident of Carmen was quite shocking, particularly since, just fifty minutes after she had left her pharmacy Carmen was seen running through a breakdown lane on I-490, near the Chili-Raga exit completely naked from waist down. The woman attempted to flee from a rear-facing Ford Pinto hatchback, waving her hands in a frantic manner at passers-by trying to draw the attention of cars passing by.

Afterward, eyewitnesses said that they had seen the dark-colored Ford slowing down toward Carmen and, within a matter of seconds, a man was seen emerging from the vehicle was seen grabbing the scared Carmen by the wrist, threw her in the car, and then sped away.

The thing that makes the story of Carmen the most heartbreaking was the incident that was witnessed by 38 people was not covered up for three days. At the time that the initial report was published Carmen's body had already been discovered just two days later by two teenagers who were almost twelve miles from the road in which she had sought assistance.

A few of her clothes would later be discovered on that same road. The 10-year-old Carmen was raped and murdered.

Could Carmen be saved if witnesses had moved swiftly enough or proceeded to pursue the suspect driving the Ford Pinto? Could she have survived If the police had been earlier notified of the tragic incident that occurred in the roadway?

Wanda Walkowicz

Age 11 years old

On April 2nd, 1973, similar to Carmen Colon, 11-year-old Wanda Walkowicz was out doing errands at the local grocery store , where she went to buy some items for her mom. According to reports, she left the house at 5:10pm. However her mother began to feel anxious when she realized that her daughter didn't return home by 8:30 after 8:00 pm. In desperation, Wanda's mother made a call to the police to make a report of her daughter's missing.

After many hours of searching, police were able to locate Wanda however not in the manner Wanda's mother might have liked. The body of Wanda was found by an New York state trooper during an inspection near Irondequoit Bay in Webster.

Although Carmen was found to be fully clothed, it was discovered that she had been an assault victim. An autopsy later revealed that Wanda was murdered by the help of the ligature.

Authorities were in confusion after the autopsy report indicated that Wanda was a custard drinker prior to when she died. The report prompted speculation that the murderer had given custard to Wanda at the time of their conversation.

Wanda's mother claimed that custard wasn't on the list of things her daughter bought at the store, and that she never was served custard in her home or at school.

In the nick of time, a reward of $10,000 was announced to anyone who could provide information that would result in an arrest of the perpetrator. Within a short time, the phone calls began flooding in. One caller claimed to have witnessed Wanda conversing with the owner of the brown vehicle located in a spot that was only 0.2 miles from her house.

Another caller said she saw a woman with hair of red that matched Wanda's description getting pushed into the light-colored Dodge vehicle by the driver. According to the witness the incident occurred between 5:30 to 6:00 midnight on the evening that Wanda disappeared.

Michelle Maenza

Age 11 years old

Michelle Maenza would end up as the final victim of the Alphabet Killer, seven months after the murder of Wanda Walkowicz. Michelle was declared missing as she returned from school on 26th November 1973.

Michelle was said to have made an excursion to an outlet store while returning home the following afternoon. The girl was reportedly there to get a purse that her mother had left there earlier.

Michelle's uncle said that he'd approached Michelle in his vehicle and offered her a ride, but Michelle declined.

At around 3:00 pm Michelle was observed by a person who was witnessing the incident to have taken a ride in a car described as being beige or tan in Ackerman Street. The girl appeared to be crying all the duration of the.

Michelle's mother later discovered her daughter was missing in a panic. There were reports from eyewitnesses that a woman who fit Michelle's description was seen at around 4:30 pm in an eatery that serves fast food with an Caucasian male. The Caucasian male was believed to be between 25-35.

Another witness who was a driver who saw the car with a tan color at around 5:30 that same day. The vehicle had an unflat tire, and also recalled having seen a woman who was similar to Michelle's description, looking like she was in a state of pain.

The driver claimed that a man seated near the car with a tan color was holding the child with his wrist. The driver also stated that he attempted to stop and examine the girl, however, he encountered quite a frightful opposition from the man who attempted to cover the girl's face behind his back while trying to hinder the license plate of his. At some point, the resistance from the person was so threatening that it frightened motorists away of the area.

Michelle's body was discovered the next day with bruises and abrasions condition, less than 15 miles from her house. Michelle as Wanda was dressed in full but the evidence that indicated sexual abuse were severe. Michelle's autopsy findings showed that she also died of strangulation by a rope, and that she was fed hamburger, which was confirmed by the account of the person who claimed to have seen her in an eatery that served fast food.

Modus Operandi

After the deaths of one or more victims is evident how his killer, the Alphabet Serial Killer has a attraction for girls in the teen years who were all said to come of Catholic families.

The murderer has been reported to be able to capture these young girls as they went out without supervision by an adult. The kids were reported to be able to enter the vehicle with ease, raising the question of whether the person who killed them was one whom the girls were acquainted with. Perhaps, he got the innocents into his car without having to fight.

Based on the police reports, it's believed that all of victims came from families with no fathers in the home. Their mothers were in welfare. It could be that this is the reason why food was a convenient way to soothe them. But it is not forgotten the fact that Wanda as well as Michelle had both been mentally disabled this could explain why they did not attempt to escape, as Carmen did.

According to autopsy findings the killer fed his victims prior to or after assaulting them sexually. Then the killer was able to strangle his victims, before dissolving their bodies.

There is an incredibly remarkable resemblance in their names, which resulted in the nickname that was given to the murderer. All of them were thrown away in a town with the same initials and names. Carmen Colon had been dumped in Churchville, Wanda Walkowicz had been thrown out in Webster while Michelle Maenza was dumped in Macedon.

Some suggested that it could be a simple coincidence, however evidence has indicated that the murderer's actions being deliberate.

Investigation

In the course of the investigation, a number of investigators believed there was a chance Carmen was killed through a person she was acquainted with. They also were of the view the possibility that Michelle and Wanda might have been killed with the help of the same individual because they were both fed, but Carmen was not.

The investigators also discovered a resemblance in Michelle and Wanda which Carmen didn't have. Both girls had hairy cat fur on them which led the police to believe that the murderer may have lured the girls by using a cat, and then made them feel at ease in his presence.

Robert Ressler, a member of the FBI Behavioural Science Unit, made an account of the murderer and also thought that Carmen's killer may be different from the killer from Wanda or Michelle.

According Robert Robert, the murderer of Carmen was known to have displayed actions of extreme anger. This could be due to Carmen's escape attempt. Additionally unlike the other victims, Carmen had no food in her stomach. It is possible that the murderer could be learning from the mistakes with carmen, and realized that feeding the girls could be an effective method to keep them in a calm state.

As the investigation continued during the investigation, a firefighter from Rochester attempted to raped an teen girl in a garage on the 1st January 1974. The man, a firefighter named Dennis Termini, was chased by the police who intervened. later Termini fired a gun when his pursuit was interrupted by policemen, and then fired his gun at himself.

The police later found out that Termini also raped a youngster at the time in the garage. Despite the fact that both teenager victims were older that those of the Alphabet Murder victims, evidence confirmed the views of policemen that Termini is a top suspect.

The car that was driven by Termini matched what was described as the car that was observed by an eyewitness, and there was a map on the vehicle that showed Wayne County. Termini was the primary suspect for decades , and in 2007 the police were permitted to test the theory when they exhumed his body.

Suspects

In each case there were suspects arrested each time, and

dismissed. When it came to Carmen there was a fascinating event had transpired that led the investigators to wonder whether the case of Carmen was actually separated from the other two girls.

Miguel Colon

In situations like the one that Carmen was in incident, it's not unusual for police to search out relatives that are victims' families first. In the wake of an eyewitness account that stated that Carmen was in the vehicle of her attacker It didn't take much time for the police to begin examining Miguel Colon.

Uncle Miguel who Carmen loved to call him, was quickly taken into custody by the police to be questioned about the disappearance of Carmen. According to reports, Miguel was more close to Carmen as well as her mother following the separation of her parents.

According to the statements made, Carmen was usually escorted to the pharmacy by her grandfather Felix. On the morning of her abduction Carmen was able get her father to allow her to leave on her own. Did this happen because someone ordered her to go on her own?

Eyewitnesses claimed they observed Carmen getting into the deep Ford Pinto, the same car she was running away from in the middle of the highway. In a strange coincidence, it was exactly the same vehicle that her uncle Miguel had just purchased. The police were prompted to investigate the vehicle and the results were possibly another indication that Uncle Miguel could be the one responsible for missing his daughter.

After searching the vehicle at Miguel's residence, officers discovered that the entire vehicle had been thoroughly cleaned with powerful cleaning solutions, including the truck. The investigators noticed that it was rare for anyone to wash your trunk vehicles as thoroughly as Miguel haddone, which raised suspicions.

Police also discovered the doll belonging to Carmen in the vehicle. However, when they asked about it Miguel dismissed the doll by saying that it had been found as a result of being a close family member and a close friend to the child. The story said that Miguel was reportedly very angry the following day, two days following Carmen was found dead. He allegedly informed one of his friends that he was required to go to Puerto Rico because he had committed an act of violence in Rochester.

In a shocking twist of events, Miguel committed suicide by self-inflicted fatal gunshots on the island of Puerto Rico. Although Miguel seemed quite guilty however, the police hadn't tried to indict or prosecute him with his murder. Carmen.

Dennis Termini

One of the prime suspects for years was a 25-year-old Rochester firefighter. Termini was also known for his track record of having been a serial rapist using the name "Garage Rapist". He was responsible for at least 14 rapes on teenage girls and women between 1971 between 1971 and 1973.

Termini was the owner of a car in a beige color and was close to Carmen Colon. According to the report, Termini killed himself after being pursued by policemen in an attempt to rape a girl within five weeks of Michelle's murder. Michelle.

After conducting a forensic investigation of the vehicle of Termini the police discovered traces of fur from a white cat that was in line with the evidence gathered from the murders of three girls.

Following the exhumation and exhumation of the Termini's corpse in 2007, the results of DNA tests revealed that he wasn't in charge of Wanda's murder. Wanda. But, there was no DNA sample of Michelle as well as Carmen which could serve to compare them.

Joseph Naso

Joseph Naso, who was an ex-photographer was arrested in the year the year 2011 in Reno. The 77-year old was accused of four counts of murder of females who were killed in California between 1977 between 1994 and 1977. Joseph Naso was known to be stalking, sexually assaulting and then put his victims in sexual poses in front of the mannequins. The victims were believed as prostitutes.

Joseph Naso became a suspect when it was revealed that his victims were carrying the same letters as their last names and their initials. The second woman Naso murdered at the hands of California was a woman aged 22 named Carmen Colon, a rather bizarre coincidence.

Police also discovered that Naso was living in Rochester in the 1970s, in the early 1970s, where he worked as a photographer for hire. Following DNA tests, the police finally proved that Naso was not the one responsible to the death of three young victims and was simply one of the copycats with a personal stake regarding The Alphabet Murders.

Kenneth Bianchi

In Rochester, New York, Kenneth was the epitomized of a troubled childhood as well as delinquency prior to his move into Los Angeles to live with his cousin at 26.

Alongside Bianchi's cousin Angelo Buono Jr., Bianchi was a one of the group known by many as"the Hillside Stranglers. They were in charge of the killings of ten teenage girls and females from Los Angeles between January 1976 between January 1976 and 1978. The victims were between 12 and 28 years old.

Kenneth was an ice cream vendor in Rochester during the time during which the murders were committed. He was also famous for driving a vehicle which was of the same color and model as the car that was seen by eyewitnesses at an abduction locations.

Police discovered evidence of forensics at the scene of the crime at which the murder of Wanda took place. The forensic evidence was believed to be found in 20 percent of males according to the way destiny would have it, Kenneth was in the 20% group. It appears as if the police had located their man.

An investigation of Kenneth through the use of a wristprint that police obtained following the death of Michelle Maenza, sadly did not correspond to Kenneth's. The man was released from the leash. There was no evidence to establish Kenneth as the murderer of Michelle.

Kenneth like everyone else has did not deny ever having anything to do with have anything to do with any of Alphabet Murders.

Conspiracy Theories

Many people believe that Kenneth Bianchi was not smart enough to be able to pull from his infamous Alphabetic Murders and got away from it.

There are those who would add that the perpetrator could be working for the institution, possibly an employee of the school, or a driver who knew that the girls been mentally handicapped. It is also possible that the girls would have been willing to travel with the person who killed them because they recognized the person. There are speculations that the perpetrator left his victims in a place at a place where they could be discovered swiftly because he probably was ashamed after having committed the crime.

Some believe that the killer may have been employed in Social Services which may have provided him with access to the records, and thus the ability to choose and take his victims as he wanted.

There is also the possibility that the killer halted his murder spree following the first three victims as they had just relocated out of the region to another location or maybe the killer was imprisoned somewhere else or perhaps he had died.

The consequences

Carmen's kidnapping was immediately condemned by the general public after it was reported in the media. Many newspapers like The Times Union and the Democrat and Chronicle immediately offered an amount of $2,500 for any information that leads to the conviction and arrest of the murderer.

Posters and billboards were put up in every corner of Rochester following the killing of Carmen Colon had occurred. There was also a massive anger and shame in Rochester over the eyewitnesses who did not do anything to assist the poor girl who was trying to get assistance, but also did not take the initiative to inform the police about the incident.

Additionally to the reward of $2,500 that was offered by Rochester local newspapers Local businesses also raised the amount of $6,000 to reward anyone who might assist with the capture of the murderer.

Many residents of Rochester at the time stated that the city had transformed into a scary city to reside in.

Chapter 4: Highway of Tears

The location: Highway 16, British Columbia, Canada

Time Frame: 1989 - 2006.

Victims: 27

WIf one is thinking of Canada when one thinks of Canada, images of tranquility, peace, and unspoiled nature will most likely pop into the mind. Canadians are recognized as being a serene, kind and accommodating group of people. That is why , when the word spread that a serial killer was believed to be in the wild and it caused anxiety through the whole nation.

The highway 16 within British Colombia had found itself to be a 450 mile-long memorial of desperation and death for Canadians in which young women started to appear dead along the road.

The highway connects both cities, Prince Rupert and Prince George. However, on the stretch of highway 16 are numerous First Nations, which are the homes of several aboriginal groups. Because of their locations, the lack of public transportation within the area and poverty, these communities are separated from both cities. The term "Highway of Tears" was created as a result of the struggle and suffering that the indigenous peoples of Canada who lived in the region.

It was noted that hitchhikers are the most at risk on Highway 16. Many drivers, including those who were also known to be indigenous took the route due to need due to the absence of public transportation and eventually became victims.

Murders

The struggles of the indigenous people are far too immense to count but the most significant tragedy is centered in the area of Highway 16, where over half of the women who vanished in mysterious ways were First Nations.

Some of them weren't heard from again, however others were discovered in the months or years that followed their disappearances, though dead. The majority of victims of the Highway 16 killings were known to be involved in the sex industry and others were hitchhikers.

Gloria Moody

Age 26 years old

Gloria Moody has been regarded as the first person to be identified as a victims of The Highway 16 killings. Her last sighting was leaving at a pub located in William's Lake, B.C. on the night of the 25th of October on the night of October 25th, 1969. Gloria was believed to be on a weekend getaway with her family when the two of them gone to several establishments on the night.

Gloria's brother said that he believed his sister was following him , and he could not recall what transpired following. The next day, after her disappearance Gloria's body was discovered on a cattle trail six miles of William's Lake by two hunters.

Gloria was battered, naked, bruised and sexually assaulted, before she passed out because of her horrific injuries.

Gale Ann Weys

Age 19 years old

Gale has been last observed at the station she worked at in Clearwater on 19th October 1973. Police believed that Gale was a hitchhiker across Clearwater to Kamloops in Kamloops, where she was living. It wasn't until one year later on the 6th day of April 1974 that her body was discovered in a flooded ditch to the south of Clearwater.

Micheline Pare

Age 18 years old

One of the last times anyone was able to see Micheline took place on Highway 29 in July 1970. According to reports, she was on her way to Quebec and was traveling by hitchhiking throughout the region. There was also a report that two women had offered Micheline an ride before dropping her off at Tompkins Ranch.

Just a few days later, on August 8, 1970 Micheline's body was discovered in Hudson's Hope. Similar to Gloria, Micheline had been sexually assaulted and beat to death by the use of a blunt object.

Pamela Darlington

Age 19 years old

Within a month of Gale Ann Weys' disappearance, Pamela Darlington had gone missing. Pamela disappeared from her favorite pub, the David Thompson Pub at the end of the day on November 6, 1973. The news reported that Pamela was seen leaving the bar with an unidentified person who had messy hair.

Frank Almon Sr. and his son found the body of Pamela one day later, near the front of their property that bordered Pioneer Park.

In the course of an investigation it was discovered that the blonde-haired male which Pamela disappeared was believed to be the driver of a white model Chrysler that was spotted by a train driver who was in the area. It was discovered that the vehicle had been trying to block trains in the region where the body of Pamela's was discovered.

Colleen MacMillen

Age 16 years old

Colleen MacMillen, who grew up at Lac La Hache with her family, was described as a shy , but friendly girl. Colleen was regarded as a reliable young lady and had a calm, steady personality.

On the 9th August 1974 The girl was just 9 years old and had planned to travel by hitchhike to a friend's home that was located only 4 miles from her home. But, Colleen only made it to Highway 97 and then disappeared.

The following month, Colleen's body was discovered in the logging home located 15 miles to the south to 100 Mile House. In addition, 100 Mile House was again 28 miles to the south of the spot the spot where Colleen was last seen.

Monica Andrea Cathy Ignas

Age 14 years old

Monica is believed to be returning back to class on the date she went missing in December 1974. Monica was last observed walking along Highway 16 and was walking towards Thornhill, B.C. before she disappeared.

The following year on the 6th day of April in 1795, Monica's corpse was discovered in a thickly wooded region at Terrance. The reason for her death was been strangulation.

Monica Jack

Age 12 years old

Monica was on her bicycle in May 1978 when she last saw at the home of her maternal grandmother. As per her mom she offered Monica an aid, however Monica insisted she would like to complete the journey by herself.

In the final analysis the only thing that was that was left from Monica was her bicycle. It was only 20 years after that her remains were discovered in a ravine, by forest workers. The ravine was 12 miles from the place where Monica disappeared.

The list of victims of the Highway 16 murders is seemingly inexhaustible. While authorities have stated that there were 27 victims Indigenous people living on the Highway 16 claimed that the government tried to cover it by claiming that there were at most 40 women murdered in the murders.

Other victims are:

* Helen Claire Frost -- 15 missing in Prince George, October 1970

* Jean Virginia Samuel18 - Missing from Hazelton Oct. 1971

* Mary Jane Hill -- 31, killed by Prince Rupert, March 1978

* Maureen Mosie -- 33, Murdered near Salmon Arm, May 1981

* Jean May Kovacs -- 36, killed by Prince George, October 1981

* Roswitha Fuchsbichler - 13 - Murdered by Prince George, November 1981

* Nina Marie Joseph -- 15, murdered in Prince George, August 1982

* Shelley-Anne Bascu - 16, missing from Hinton in May 1983.

* Alberta Gail Williams -- 24, killed close to Prince Rupert, August 1989

* Cecilia Anne Nikal -- 15 missing from Smithers in October, 1989.

* Delphine Anne Nikal 15, missing from Smithers June 1990

* Theresa Umphrey -- 38 -- Murdered close to Prince George, February 1993

* Marnie Blanchard - 18, murdered close to Prince George, March 1993

* Ramona Lisa Wilson 16 years old, murdered near Smithers in June 1994.

* Roxanne Thiara -- 15 years old, murdered close to Burns Lake, November 1994

* Alishia Leah Germaine 15, murdered by Prince George, November 1994

* Lana Derrick -- 19, missing from Terrace in October, 1995.

* Deena Braem - 16 killed near Quesnel on September 29, 1999.

* Monica McKay -- 18 murdered by Prince Rupert, December 1999

* Nicole Hoar -- 24 missing in Prince George, June 2002

* Mary Madeline George -- 25, missing From Prince George, July 2005

* Tamara Lynn Chipman -- 22, missing From Prince Rupert, September 2005

* Aielah Saric Auger 14 - Murdered in Prince George, February 2006

* Beverly Warbick -- 20 missing From Prince George, June 2007

* Bonnie Marie Joseph -- 32, Missing from Vanderhoof, September 2007

* Jill Stacey Stuchenko -- 35, killed close to Prince George, October 2009

* Emmalee Rose McLean -- 16 years old. Murdered in Prince Rupert, April 2010

* Natasha Lynn Montgomery -- 23rd murder by Prince George, August 2010

* Cynthia Frances Maas-- 35, murdered close to Prince George, September 2010

* Loren Dawn Leslie 15, murdered near Prince George, November 2010

* Madison "Maddy" Scott -- 20, Missing near Vanderhoof, May 2011

* Immaculate "Mackie" Basil -26, missing close to Fort St. James, June 2013,

* Anita Florence Thorne -- 49, missing From Prince George, November 2014

* Roberta Marie Sims -- 55, missing From Prince George, May 2017

* Frances Brown -- 53 Missing near Smithers on October 17, 2017

* Chantelle Catherine Simpson 34, Suspicious Death on Terrace in July of 2018

* Jessica Patrick -- 18 Murdered near Smithers in September of 2018

* Cynthia Martin -- 50, Missing near Hazelton, December 2018

Modus Operandi

It is interesting that the Highway 16 killings seem to exclusively target female victims However, one thing that makes this M.O. extra distinctive was the way the murderer displayed a preference to indigenous women.

Highway 16 murderer Highway 16 murderer would abduct his victims, assault them sexually them, then end their lives by the method of strangulation in the majority of instances, or by beating them to death.

Investigation

The rise in murders that remain unsolved and disappearances of women on Highway 16 has put the spotlight off B.C. and Canadian news and sparked the attention and interest of the local, national as well as international scales.

There was a consistent pattern of starting and ending the investigation that led to the Highway 16 killings. This led to possibility that the murderer could have been detained repeatedly between murders.

The investigators also were of the view that there several serial murderers in the area. in the region. The theory was substantiated after a number of people were found guilty of murders that took place along Highway 16.

The RCMP initiated a provincially funded project in 2005 dubbed E-Pana. The purpose of the project was to concentrate on unsolved murders and disappearances that happened in the vicinity of Highway 16.

One of the main goals of the project was to determine if the murders along Highway 16 were the work of one serial killer , or the aftermath of multiple murderers who picked this highway for their site of preference.

E-Pana began with three cases in 2005. In two years it was reached 18. E-Pana used a set of criteria to screen victims. They only took in those who were females, who have a track record of hitchhiking and known for being associated with commercial sexual work, and located near Highway 16, Highway 97 as well as Highway 5 at the time of their disappearance or at the time their bodies were discovered.

The E-Pana project was acknowledged as having the connection to Colleen MacMillen's death to Bobby Jack Fowler. The project also succeeded in bringing the murder charge against Garry Taylor Handlen for the murder of Monica Jack in 1978. Handlen is found guilty the year 2019 and sentenced to life imprisonment this was the first ever case that was officially resolved which included a court hearing and a sentenced suspect.

The E-Pana project is currently operating, examining the remaining instances that are part of the Highway of Tears.

Suspects

Many suspects were arrested during the investigation. Many of them already had criminal records, and others were ultimately discovered guilty for being involved in the Highway 16 murders, thanks to the evidence found that were just too grave to overlook. Here are a few suspects:

Cody Alan Legebokoff

The tragedy for Cody began when an Royal Canadian Mounted Police officer observed his truck entering an unreachable logging road along Highway 27. According to reports, the officer suspected Cody of speeding, and directed him to stop.

The officer, after being assisted by a police officer, reported that they observed blood splashed on Cody's face and chin as well as both legs. This led them to a area of blood in the floor of the his seat.

A look inside the pickup found a multi-tool as well as a wrench coated with blood. The vehicle was further searched and resulted in the discovery of the monkey's bag and the wallet contained the hospital card for children. The card's name is Loren Donn.

Cody was then interrogated about the body's blood and he claimed the poaching was in the region and murdered a deer. In the end, Cody was detained under the Canadian Wildlife Act.

Incredibly, something didn't seem to be right, the police officer traced the tracks of Cody's tire truck, and eventually led police towards the remains of Loren Donn Leslie.

Cody Legebokoff pleaded guilty of murder and was sentenced to life prison without release for more than 25 years as a result of the murders committed by four Highway 16 victims: Loren Donn Leslie, Cynthia Frances Maas, Natasha Lynn Montgomery, and Jill Stacey Stuchenko.

Cody was also believed to be among the youngest serial killers to be recorded in Canada's history. Canada.

Bobby Jack Fowler

A man with a high profil, Bobby Jack Fowler was an American rapper who performed in his native country and across the border into Canada. Fowler was an engineer and famous for his travels throughout North America.

Fowler has managed to build an arrest record throughout his travels and was convicted of numerous violent crimes that included sexual assault, attempted murder and firearm-related offences.

Fowler was found guilty of first degree kidnapping, rape in the first degree and coercion, as well as fourth-degree assault and menacing. In the end, Fowler was sentenced to prison for 16 years and would die in the month of May 2006 at approximately 66 years old from lung cancer.

The year 2012 was the time that Fowler was identified as a possible suspect in Highway 16 cases when his DNA was discovered in the remains of Colleen MacMillen. Fowler was also identified as a key candidate for murder in the cases of Pamela Darlington and Gale Weys. As per the RCMP there was a possibility that Fowler was the one responsible in the murders of up to twenty Highway 16 murder cases.

Garry Taylor Handlen

Handlen made his professional career in 1969 after the judge found him guilty of sexual assault at the age of 22. After the conviction Handlen received a sentence of six months' imprisonment.

It is possible to think that crime is similar to drugs because in the year 1971, two years later than his initial sentence, Handlen found himself in the court again. This time , the accusation against Handlen was rape, and Handlen was sentenced to five years , six months prison.

In the spirit of encyclicality, as his life allowed, Handlen picked up a passenger in a hitchhiker's path near Hope, B.C. in 1978. He then proceeded sexually attack her. Handlen was said to have taken her by the neck and choked the victim with his naked hands. Unfortunately for Handlen the victim was able to escape naked and was quickly taken away by a motorcyclist and a good Samaritan.

Handlen was found guilty of a second time for 18 years of prison, however his sentence was reduced by the Canadian Court of Appeal would reduce the punishment to 12 years.

The reports stated that Handle was keeping an unassuming presence in Edmonton after his release from prison. However, in 2014 following the examination of new forensic evidence by the police Handlen aged 66, he was arrested. of age, was charged with two murder charges in the first degree in the murders of Monica Jack and Kathryn-Mary Herbert.

Garry Taylor Handlen was found guilty by jurors and sentenced to life imprisonment for the year 2019.

Brian Peter Arp

According to court documents witnesses had witnessed Marie Blanchard enter a small grey Toyota or Nissan pickup truck following some hesitation. The driver was described as a male with black shoulder length hair, with some of his hair lying on his left side.

Marnie Blanchard's remains have been discovered by a cross-country skier about 6 miles from the city of Prince George. A review between medical documents was made in order that the police could confirm the identity of Marnie Blanchard.

On the 18th of April of 1990, police began to search the gray Nissan truck registered to the wife of Arp's common law. A double-edged knife that had four inches of blade was discovered inside the door pocket of the driver's seat, as well as an engraved silver ring hidden under the seat of the passenger. The ring was later recognized by family members of the victim as belonging to her.

The further inspection of the vehicle resulted in finding two tiny purple fibers that were found in the carpet under the passenger's seat. In this way, a portion of carpet was cut off by police, and then handed to a fiber and hair expert who determined they were compatible with the fabric that was used to create the victim's sweater.

Brian Arp was arrested the next day, charged with second-degree killing of

Marnie Blanchard. Arp later volunteered to provide samples of his scalp and hair. But, the samples were not identical to the 16 hair samples that were found within Blanchard's clothing.

The case that involved Theresa Umphrey, although Arp did not provide samples for DNA testing, police managed to take the DNA samples of his from cigarettes' butts that Arp was smoking during his time with police.

Unfortunately for Arp his DNA test, it were positive and Arp was arrested on fourth of the month, October 4, 1993 in connection with killing in the 1st degree of Theresa Umphrey and then re-arrested in connection with the first-degree killing of Marie Blanchard,

Brian Arp was found guilty by an Quesnel Jury in March 1995 for the murders of Marie Blanchard in 1989 and Theresa Umphrey in 1993. Arp was sentenced at minimum 25 years in prison prior to any chance of parole.

Conspiracy Theories

The question of race was the most popular theory to preoccupy those who were killed on the Highway 16 killings. Some critics believed that systematic racism was the primary reason the murders were not properly probed by authorities. They also argued that the media had also slowed their coverage of the case because they were of lesser importance given to women with native origin as compared to women who were not indigenous.

The argument for racial bias in the case was strengthened when Nicole Hoar, who was an Caucasian woman, went missing in 2002. Most important media outlets across the country covered the instance, in contrast to the time when Indigenous women went missing.

The consequences

The disappearances and killings of indigenous women provoked an outrage in the local community. It was revealed that the probability for the Aboriginal female to become killed during the course of her life in Canada is four-fold greater than the case of a non-native Canadian. The report suggested that race was a factor in the way these deaths were carried out.

A number of indigenous groups have made an argument that the absence of proper investigations by police was the result of prejudice based on race that sparked an uproar and an interest in cases like the Highway 16 cases.

Following the Highway 16 killings, the Highway of Tears Symposium was organized in which 33 distinct suggestions were made on how to decrease the risk of victimization throughout the region. In addition, recommendations for implementing the crime prevention program for the region were offered.

A subdued transit service began operating on Highway 16 and has lowered the risk of hitchhiking for people of poor origin and in turn, the risk level of hitchhikers within the region.

Chapter 5: Freeway Phantom

Place: Washington D.C

Time Frame 1971 to 1972

Victims: 6

The capital city of the United States became the playground of the serial killer who had an obsession with youngsters African American girls and perhaps was obsessed with taking their shoes off. What is the reason anyone would do that? One might wonder. However, the time that serial killers began to actually make any sense to a brain?

Murders

The Freeway Phantom had managed to take the lives of six innocent children in two years with no consequences. Who were the girls who's life was cut off in such a way and abruptly?

Carol Spinks

Age 13 years old

Carol Spinks was regarded as the first victim of the Freeway Phantom. Carol was twin, and was among the eight children that disappeared on April 25, 1971. Carol was a child who had gone missing to avoid her mother's order not to leave home and at the request by her sister.

Carol's mother noticed her along the way and instructed her daughter to head straight to her home and she never made her return.

Carol's body was discovered after six days on I-295. The girl was dressed, but her shoes were not to be seen. The autopsy report stated that she had died for about two to three days prior to her discovery. The fruit of citrus was discovered in Carol's stomach. This indicated that her killer been feeding her during the time he held her hostage in a cell for several days prior to her death.

Darlenia Johnson

Age 16 years old

Darlenia Johnson became the victim number two of Darlenia Johnson was the second victim of Freeway Phantom. On July 9, 1971 Darlenia had been reported missing because she had not turned into the Recreation Center where she worked.

Two witnesses claimed that they had observed Darlenia prior to her disappearance. One witness claimed they saw Darlenia along with her lover and the other said they had observed her and an unknown African American man. The leads from both bear no fruit.

11 days following her abduction Darlenia's body was discovered on I-295 by an D.C. Department of Highways and Traffic employee, which was just 15 feet from the spot the spot where Carol Spinks' body had been discovered. There was no evidence to support this case Darlenia due to the extreme decomposition the body went through due to the high humidity and heat levels. Similar to Carol Darlenia's shoe, Darlenia's was not found.

Brenda Crockett

Age 10 years old

Brenda was the third victim and youngest from the Freeway Phantom. Brenda was sent for an errand the 27th July 1971.

Brenda's mother escorted her out around 8:00pm believing that her daughter had brought a friend along. Brenda left the house in bare feet with a pink curler, but was taken as she headed to the Safeway to purchase bread and food for her family pets.

After an hour of her not coming home to her family, the mom went out to find her, while her 7-year-old sister left her home. Brenda was said to have called her home around 9:20 pm, and informed the younger sibling that she was taken by a white man from Virginia and was returning in a cab. Brenda's sister also said that she was crying throughout the entire time she was talking to her via the phone.

After a short time, Brenda was reported to have called her home again, but the call was returned to her mother's boyfriend. Brenda simply repeated the same thing she said during the previous phone call, and the boyfriend asked whether Brenda had any idea of the area she was in Virginia.

Brenda responded "No," then added, "Did my mother see me?"

The boyfriend of her mother was puzzled by this query and inquired about how Brenda's mother would have seen her if she had been in Virginia.

To try to comprehend the situation the boyfriend asked Brenda to place her abductor's name to the telephone. She simply replied with the words "I'll be back." before closing the call.

Contrary to the two previous instances where the bodies of victims was discovered after couple of days, Brenda's body was found by a hitchhiker along Route 50 the next day. Because of the time within which Brenda's body was discovered, it was clear what was happening to her. Brenda was sexually assaulted, and a green scarf that she was wearing put on by her murderer in order to choke her.

Nenomoshia Yates

Age 12 years old

Nenomoshia was sent for an errand at the nearby Safeway store on the 1st day of October 1971. The date on which Nenomoshia got to the store remains unclear. According to reports from a witness, that Nenomoshia was seen entering the blue Volkswagen.

Nenomoshia was discovered the same day on Pennsylvania Avenue in Prince

George's County, Maryland. The remains were still warm when it was discovered, meaning that she was dead for a couple of hours , if not more. Sixteen-year-old girl was brutally raped and killed. Green synthetic fibers that were not identified were also discovered on her clothes.

Similar to the two previous victims, the shoes of Nenomoshia were not found.

Brenda Woodard

Age 18 years old

Brenda Woodard had been out with her friends on the 15th November 1971. But, Brenda split from her group after she moved buses.

A little over six hours later, when Brenda disappeared her body was discovered just off Route 202.

In the same way as Brenda Crockett and Nenomoshia Yates, Brenda Woodard had also been brutally assaulted and taken hostage in the hands of her kidnapper. However, the abductor took it one step further by stabbing her four times.

The murderer also left an unmarked note in Brenda's pockets. The note was written written by Brenda, however the writing was that of the murderer. Here's what was written in the document:

"this is akin to my sensitivity to females, particularly. I'll be honest with you in the event that you catch me, when you can! Free-way Phantom!"

The speculation is that Brenda may have been aware of the murderer since the note was written in her usual writing style, without any evidence of desperation. The police also believe that Brenda was in an argument after being stabbed in the back by the kidnapper. This was supported through the defensive injuries found on her body that indicated there was a fight.

Brenda Woodard was the oldest victim of the Freeway Phantom.

Diane Williams

Age 17 years old

Diane Williams had gone missing on September 5, 1972. The gap between dates was thought to be significant since it had been more than 10 months after the murderer was active.

The boyfriend of Diane was the last to meet her at around 10:30 pm on the day that they took her back to her bus stop. Her body was found several hours later on I-295 which brought us back to the exact spot that the murderer put his first set of victims.

While Diane was also in a similar way to other victims but she was not sexually assaulted, and her white sneakers were also found along with her.

Modus Operandi

The Freeway Phantom was known to target women African American children and teenagers. The victims fell within the age group between 10 and 18 years old. The serial killer used to follow the habit of abducting his victims as they went about their daily routine to run errands or returning from work. The killer would then assault his victims, taking them to the grave through strangulation before dropping them in grassy areas around freeways. This led to the moniker "Freeway Phantom".

Perhaps, taking cues of the Long Island Killer, the Freeway Phantom did not follow his usual pattern when it came to his third victim. He forced her to contact her family two times, which could be seen as an attempt to annoy the family of the victim as well as cause confusion for the police.

The Freeway Phantom was also adept at collecting memorabilia from his victims. The killer kept a journal as well as curlers and shoelaces of three victims.

Investigation

Since the start of the killings in the year 1971 the mystery of Freeway Phantom had been one that investigators struggled to resolve. The murders were stopped 17 months after the beginning of the murders.

In the course of the investigation, a variety of information was received from the general public via an anonymous hotline run through MPDC. Metropolitan Police Department of the District of Columbia (MPDC). The investigation was conducted by a department of law enforcement, which included police officers from Prince Georges County and Montgomery County, Maryland, detectives from the MPDC Homicide department, Maryland state police and the FBI.

In the context of the time that detectives who were assigned to the case were responsible of the case file at the MPDC Detective Division, some of the documents and notes in those files were lost, as well as others being removed completely. This led to being unable to access the Freeway Phantom case files being in a state of utter disarray.

Though the majority of the investigators who are assigned on the case retired or have passed away however, the Freeway Phantom remains an active case to present within the MPDC Homicide Division.

Suspects

No matter how many instances that police received information and clues but there was still no definitive suspect in the case, and nobody had been caught by police. The suspects included:

Green Vega Rapists

The Green Vega Rapists had already been extensively investigated as the main suspected suspects in the Freeway Phantom cases. In the course for the probe, each person in the band was detained within Lorton Prison in Virginia, where they were serving prison sentences for the offenses they were convicted of previously in their home state of D.C. area previously.

In the course of the interview during the interviews, one of the imprisoned group members from the Green Vega Rapists claimed to have information regarding The Freeway Phantom killings under the requirement that his identity remain secret. The prisoner in question was able to inform the police of the dates and the locations of one of the murders . He even provided an "signature" that was not available to the general public.

Because of his intimate knowledge of the crime The police were forced to decide if there was any involvement as a suspect in this homicide. Freeway Phantom homicides. However, he was later removed from suspicion based on an excuse he offered.

It appeared that the police were going to be able to make progress in the investigation, but the lead ended up being ruined when one of the presidential candidates for the Maryland elections made public announcements they had received crucial data from an inmate in Lorton Prison regarding the Freeway Phantom case.

As if he was worried about his identity, the prisoner was reluctant to provide further details to investigators. He even went so to deny that he had ever spoken to investigators in the first place. The retraction was an enormous setback to the investigation.

Robert Elwood Askins

In March 1997 Askins worked as a technician for computers was accused of abducting and rape of a young woman at his residence. After being interrogated the police discovered that Atkins was previously convicted for other criminal acts.

Many decades prior, the time Atkins was a teenager 19 years old, he served cyanide-laced whiskey to five prostitutes in an establishment in

1938. The result was that one prostitute Ruth McDonald died.

Just two days after the death of Ruth McDonald, Atkins stabbed another prostitute to death in the brothel. Atkins was swiftly arrested and he confessed during interrogation the fact that he had been a "woman hater'. Authorities immediately put Atkins under mental surveillance.

A violent and violent person, Atkins was made to be freed when he was under observation for mental illness and assaulted three employees in the facility prior to when being detained. Atkins was found insane and placed in St. Elizabeth's hospital.

After his release at the end of April in 1952 Atkins committed murder on a woman aged 42 just five months afterward. Atkins was arrested at the time of his trial in 1954. He was tried again for the crime occurred in 1938. It was determined that Atkins was mentally stable when the murder took place and was found guilty of second degree murder and given a sentence of 20 years prison.

But, Atkins' 20-year sentence was rescinded in 1958.

Atkins was approached in prison about his involvement in the Freeway Phantom while serving time for two abductions and a rape in the D.C region. Atkins has denied involvement in the murders. He is reported to have claimed that he did not possess the mental morality necessary to be able to commit these Freeway Phantom crimes.

Because of his prior involvement associated with St. Elizabeth's Hospital, certain investigators believed that Atkins might have been involved in the murders of those six girls, however there no evidence to connect the man with the murders.

Atkin was later to die in prison at 91 after serving his sentence for two charges of abduction and rape.

Edward Sullivan and Tommie Simmons

While little information regarding these two men is readily available, Edward Sullivan and Tommie Simmons were policemen who were detained in relation with the murder of Angela Denise Barnes.

During the investigation Angela was thought as one of those who were victims in that Freeway Phantom case. However, it was discovered that Angela was not among the victims of serial murders and the police merely reopened investigations into Freeway Phantom crime scene.

Conspiracy Theories

As with in the Highway of Tears case, certain people believed that the murders would not have been solved had the victims been white. According to this theory the authorities had been very lenient in their handling on this Freeway Phantom case by the authorities.

The comparatively low media coverage or anger over this case was compared to cases that had victims who were white, leading to the notion that white cases were more popular than cases where blacks suffered the brunt of the attack.

"Those Black girls didn't mean nothing to anyone else that I'm talking about the department of police. If they had been white they would have put more force behind that, and that's for sure. it," claimed Tommy Musgrove who was a member of police in the D.C. police in 1972 and later was the director of the homicide squad.

"Dispatchers dispatched officers to the scene, and they radioed "10-8," which means that they'd discovered nothing, and they were moving forward. The officers didn't go out to look for remnants," Jenkins says. "They simply drove by." (Source: Grunge.com)

One week later on the 19th of July someone who had called went back to the scene and discovered bodies there, decaying in the scorching heat. Disappointed by the lack of action from officers, the person reported the incident to his boss who was driving by, saw it , and called his friend Charles Baden, a D.C. police sergeant. Baden was on leave the day of the incident. "He gave me the exact location it was located on the highway that was opposite 295 near the north end from Bolling Air Force Base," Baden, now 77 remembers. "I asked whether he had called the police and he responded"Yes, but no one did.'" Baden rode the road on his motorbike and drove on the road until he came across the body. (Source: Washington Post)

Chapter 6: Alabama: Sherry Lynn Marler

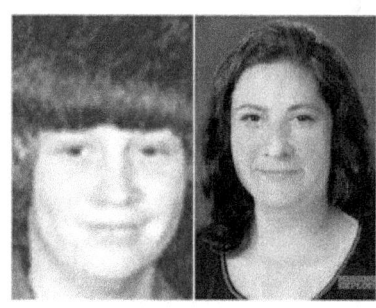

The day of June 6 1984 began similar to the Stringfellow family on their farm located in Greenville, Alabama.

Greenville which is home to the manservant, had a total population of approximately seven,600 in 1984.

The town was called camelia town after requesting that the camelia be made the official flowers for Alabama in 1959. Greenville may have provided the look of a peaceful and quiet spot to raise the morale of a family.

Betty got up early due to the fact that having to go to the Waffle House for breakfast at 7:15 a.m. in time for the

start of her shift. When she was ready
her breakfast. She then left the home.

She didn't have to wake her twelve-year
older sister, Sherry, who was asleep on
the couch at the time of she threw her
bed away to her stepdad's kinswoman ,
who was in town for the week.

When she woke up at it was 9:00 a.m.
the fortified wine identified that her
step-parent Raymond was assisting his
red van on the road.

She walked out of the housewith heels
in her hands, asking to go with him to
the city.

Around 9:15 a.m. The couple stopped
by the primary commercial bank, hoping
that Raymond could sign documents.

Fortified wine was the first thing she
needed when she was dehydrated,
therefore Raymond handed his stepchild an address and advised she
should go and get drinks at the Chevron
petrol station that is across the road. .

Witnesses reported seeing fortified wine
strolling through the parking area for
cars near the phone building as well as

Jernigan's furniture shop to an oil station.

15 minutes later, Raymond had finished at the bank and was standing to his truck, bent over.

He was shocked that the fortified wine was not there waiting to his arrival.

Another twenty-five minutes went by without any sign of the fortified wine, and panic began to set in.

Raymond is referred to by Betty on the way to Waffle House to visualize if the fortified wine was stopping by to pay a visit.

Betty identical no... Betty was the same no... was last seen by her girl the next morning, sleeping in the sofa.

Raymond tried the plain spots for his father-in-law, exactly as Chevron However, he was not so lucky.

He also contacted the store for tractor and, consequently, that's where the feed stores are located.

Her popular nickname used to be "Little Farmer" for a reason. She was a smitten girl with everything related to farming. with hanging out, get into these shops.

But nobody had ever seen any fortified wine. The woman was reported to be lost at around 11.46 a.m.

In the nick of time, a huge research project was in the making. The volunteers went around the city and its surrounding areas with an extremely fine tooth comb.

A search by air was performed with the help of Crenshaw Flying Service.

Friends, family and volunteers have printed hundreds of missing person posters and hung posters up in towns and towns in the vicinity.

Despite all the effort, Sherry remains missing.

Sherry might be Caucasian woman with brown eyes and brown hair.

When she vanished in 1984 her height was 5 feet 4 inches in height and weighted up around one hundred to twenty-pounds.

There are two marks on her body that include a 2 inch scar in her abdomen and an 1 in scar near her back. her shoulder. The fortified wine she was drinking was last seen with an oversized red fabric, light jeans, grey Velcro-fastened shoes and the watch that has an black strap.

Run away

Although it's heartbreaking, as it may be, it's unusual for children to be able to run away from their home.

In 1984, for instance in 1984, the Department of Health and Human Services disclosed to Congress on the amount of youth who were runaway within the United States was "over one million..

But did Sherry one of the millions of people who are runaways? The mother of Sherry Betty always claimed that she was a content and happy child who had no major issues.

She claimed that Sherry was not a good reason to leave the home. Sherry was thrilled about her plans for the day she went missing She was planning to catch her favourite television show and go to visit her grandmother.

Everyone was in agreement Sherry was a typical girl who did what she was instructed to do.

Also, she didn't carry anything with her when she headed to town.

Furthermore the fact that she hasn't ever contacted her family throughout the time she was gone.

Stranger abduction

The kidnapping of strangers is not common however Sherry may have been snatched by someone while walking in the park to grab an alcoholic drink.

It's not that difficult to grab someone and then pull them into your car.

Sherry may be also ripped off at the Chevron station. Her mother has pointed out that the vending machines in 1984 did not offer change.

Perhaps Sherry approached someone at the station to request change and the stranger seized the chance and abducted her.

Three sightings unconfirmed of Sherry from three different sources are also in support of the theory of abduction by strangers.

All the reports of sightings put Sherry with an individual who was believed to be in the vicinity of 50 and who was 5ft 8in tall.

He was a hoarse person and a shabby-looking appearance. One witness reported hearing the girl call him "B.J." Incredibly all three witnesses informed the police that the person that they thought was Sherry seemed extremely angry disorganized, disheveled and confused.

A person she knew was murdered

It's not surprising that Raymond Sherry's stepparent was the first person who was questioned by police.

He was the one who was the last to investigate her, in the end. Raymond worked with the police and responded to all inquiries.

However , when they asked him to undergo an instrument test for medical reasons and he declined, he said no.

In any case, the police stated that the suspect was not an suspect in the case.

His adult woman Betty believed that Raymond didn't have any hurt on his stepchild.

He never got over the reality that fortified wine was present when she vanished.

Just in the time before Raymond passed away at the end of April, 2003. He wrote an adult woman friend from her bed "Betty I'd like to know if to get some fortified wine and bring her home for you however, I am unable to do this because of I find out where she's.

If Raymond was not concerned about Sherry's disappearance. Could it be another person she was aware of?

In the year 2018, at in the Berkeley County Sheriff's workplace in South Carolina same fortified wine shared a room with her half-sister's husband and half-sister's half-sister in the St. Stephen space close to Betaw Road within the summer of 1983.

Authorities received a hint that fortified wine was observed in the same place after her disappearance in 1984.

Did these relationships have any way concerned about Sherry's disappearance?

In this case did they decide to take the wine against their will? Did fortified wine really left home and they sought protection within South Carolina for a few reasons?

In the year 2019 there was a impressive article on fortified wines Lynn Marler's still missing Facebook page.

A woman identified as Ryan Welch Anderson same she as a gang of volunteers had scoured the streets for years to find out the history of fortified wines.

They must be able to prove that they are not going to remain in their own world any longer. A portion of their message is:

Sherry Marler was killed and dismembered by a person who she was familiar with o.k. not her stepfather, and thrown into an extremely pigpen located in pantryman County.

We're inclined to believe that the one who died is dead. We are inclined to strongly believe that there may have been one or two other people during the time of his death, who are also dead.

We have a strong suspicion that she was expecting at the time.

We suspect that she was a victims of an multi-family, illegal carnal knowledge paraphilia network that included people from the pantryman and Crenshaw counties.

Ryan claims they found an old pig farm which was operating in 1984, but was abandoned and turned over to nature.

The group claims to have footage of two distinct teams of cadaver dog teams that have confirmed that human remains were beaten within the region.

While digging they found clothing which were sent to DNA tests.

It was reported that the Greenville Police Department said no DNA evidence was detected on the device.

For me, the fabric appears more like a burlap-like bag as opposed to denim or even the red plaid shirts Sherry was wearing when she vanished.

Ryan claims that a family member who survived from the man she thinks was murdered Sherry permitted her to go through an old box of photographs.

A few photographs showed the pig farm operating. One photo, in particular stunned Ryan It was a photograph of a pig sitting in front of what she claimed was a human head that had been cut off that was yet to be decomposed.

Ryan claims she took a picture of the picture using her cellphone. The original photograph was taken from her family member's home by the law enforcement agencies and handed over into the FBI.

In the end, since nothing was happening regarding the case, Ryan called the FBI and was informed they'd never seen such an image.

I find it difficult to determine exactly what's on the image This could appear to be one of the cases in which something is shaped of something you'd want to observe.

If Ryan and his team of researchers have discovered any evidence for Sherry is yet to be determined However, their dedication to the investigation and getting answers for Sherry's beloved family members cannot be doubted.

What has happened to Sherry?

Sherry was a charming romantic girl. UN agency was fond of when she was a kid, playing outdoors and keeping track of her Kenny Rogers albums.

She was a sly girl and was eager to switch her minibike into three-wheeler when she turned thirteen on her birthday.

The people she adores would have lived for decades, but they did not answering.

Everyday Betty's mother Betty faced the devastating reality the fact that one of her daughters is still to disappear.

Then her dad figure Raymond died without having any idea what happened to wine fortified.

Yet, Betty still manages to find a way to be a bit more comfortable. She declared: "Sherry has invariably been happy and contented and that's what I think about the most even in my dreams.

Betty was determined to keep the memory of her child. She inaugurated her Enterprise facility at Gregorian year VI in 2010 the 26th day of the anniversary of the disappearance of Sherry.

The check on the road mentioned earlier was "opened in memory and honor of the fortified wines Lynn Marler". Betty said, "We need to honor the memory of Lynn Marler.

We also have to create individuals who are responsive to the reality of missing kids every day across this nation.

At that point, Betty joined Team HOPE Help helping oldsters empower themselves which was a program developed in collaboration with the National Center of Missing and Exploited children to help coach the relationships of sexually exploited or missing youngsters so to assist others in their situation.

Betty stated, "At Team Hope we take care of members from the area units of a club that no one would ever want to join.

I am a volunteer in the hope that no one other person will ever endure what our family endured.

Chapter 7: COLORADO: pageant queen JonBenet Ramsey

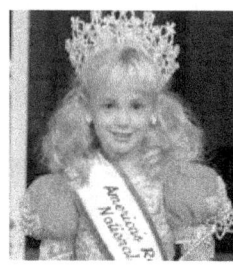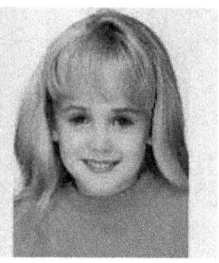

It is believed that the Colorado police detective who died in the UN agency that died from cancer in 2010, and had conducted more than two hundred investigations during his time and each one of them was a junction rectifier leading to a conviction similar to his great-grandchild Jessa van der Woerd.

She is currently being tasked along with other family members with locating her latest case, which is part of her final wish - - that of six-year-old JonBenet Ramsey.

After he was diagnosed of cancer... He knew his time was limited and, at the time, the doctor would talk to him about not being a part of this particular case. dying," the same Cindy Marra, Smit's girl. "It was vital for Smit.

As part of their pledge to keep the case going, van der Woerd and Smit's alternate great-grandchild Lexi Marra, has developed the audio podcast "The The Victim's Shoes" where they talk about the key issues of the case.

Smit was named retired to assist the investigation for three months after JonBenet was discovered dead in the basement area of the family house located in Boulder, Colo.

In the early dawn of Gregorian calendar month 26 in 1996, he was discovered dead in the basement area of the parents' home in Boulder, Colo. found only an hour later.

JonBenet is discovered dead in the basement of her parents.

JonBenet's parents initially believed that they had kidnapped her overnight.

While at work, 911, at about six in the morning Her mom, Mark Ramsey, was distraught as she told the dispatcher that her child was missing. She also found a ransom note in the at the bottom of her stairs.

The three-page document stated in part that, if the JonBenet citizens made contact with the authorities, she'd be killed and demanded $118,000.

JonBenet's parents would get an answer from the alleged of criminal "tomorrow" at 8am until 10am.

It was horrible," John Ramsey told ABC's News "Barbara Walters" in the year 2000.

In the beginning, we don't want to determine if the criminal was poised to make the decision due to the nature it was not mentioned in the document. As mentioned " I'm asking you to make a decision the next day.

Take your time and get plenty of sleep. I would get anxious that tomorrow could be the day of the twenty-seventh. ""You are lost in the time, where you are," Ramsey added in 2000. "

You've received a devastating and crushing blow. Police arrived just after the 911 call and began to investigate the scene to find clues about the suspect.

But, with the Ramsey's friends being on hand to provide moral support, they caused a sour taste by driving to home.

Police did a poor job in securing the incident... And If you don't secure this site, you'll never get an evidence that is credible," said Diane Dimond who is an associate degree investigator within the United Nations United Nations. United Nations.

. "People were thronging around the house that was being built at the moment. They were in the room they were in the front room, and there were relatives of Patsy's who were there to help her tidy the room.

There could be fingerprints on the floor. After several hours police began to remove themselves from Ramsey's home.

The residents of JonBenet were anxiously waiting for the verdict of the suspected criminal, with only one detective present: Linda Arndt.

After ten in morning and no conclusion, Arndt said that "none of JonBenet's citizens knew" the fact that "the deadline set by the requester to pay ransom"[had] vanished ".

Arndt was able to instruct John Ramsey to go and examine the house to find any indication that his daughter's possessions weren't in the right place. He discovered JonBenet at the bottom area, which was part of the house , which the police had not looked for.

I immediately knew what I'd discovered. I discovered my female offspring "John Ramsey" told Walters that he had told Walters in the year 2000. " She lay on the floor on a white blanket.

She was wrapped in a blanket. The hands of the man were tied over his head. The woman had duct tape on her mouth. ...

I immediately knelt on her and rubbed her cheek, then straightaway pulled the tape out of her mouth.

I tried to unravel the twine around his arms but couldn't untie the knot. John Ramsey aforementioned he brought his daughter upstairs and placed her down on the ground in the hope that she would be alive. Arndt informed him the girl was dead.

Arndt at the time of the incident expressed her worry that JonBenet's father was responsible for the death of their daughter, so she rehearsed herself for a possible confrontation.

We tend to check out each other I keep in mind I was wearing a holster placing my gun next to Maine and conscious of tally that I have even 18 bullets." Arndt aforementioned, adding: "

I didn't. I don't understand how we were all alive after people came to the scene.

JonBenet's cause of the death was determined to be strangulation using the aid of a bandage made from which in the case involved an untied string that was wrapped around one of Ramsey's paintbrushes.

The child also suffered an 8-inch bone fracture, shock to an arm and an offence that is regulated using a piece of applicator that was used within the bandage. This is in line the report of Brad Garrett, a former federal agent as well as CBS' News contributor. UN agency was not involved in JonBenet's situation.

JonBenet's murder JonBenet occurred on the heels of the murder of O.J. Simson and soon gained attention in the media around the world. The case is currently being discussed, police were keen to inquire about JonBenet's former associates.

Particularly after starting with children of this age and they die, they're more likely to be killed in the arms of elders," Garrett told "20/20". "So the primary target could naturally be the elderly initially, but if they're in the house. The ransom note is made on a pad that belongs to the chump.

Police began to think that the Ramseys were the ones who "harmed their son in some way or in another way, and then they panic-struck and attempted to cause seizures.

There are reasons to believe that it was. The three-page ransom note for instance was written on a Ramsey's chump pad using the pen of a household.

The amount of $118,000 was also a bit suspicious for authorities.

If you think about that range and how relevant that it's... John Ramsey was awarded a bonus by his employer for the sum of 118,000 dollars." the same Garrett who made reference to JonBenet's father.

How many of us know that? I am beginning to think that there aren't all of us "Garrett like.

JonBenet's son of John Ramsey, his twin brother John Saint Andrew Ramsey, same family that gave fingerprints and blood to police as element of the investigation.

But the rebuke of JonBenet's oldersters are the most suspects in the current investigation during formal interrogation by the police station proved problematic.

Police... will be in a battle with lawyers and wealthy friends. People from the group United Nations agency notify the police, "Give them room".

They're grieving about the situation, the same Dimond. Police believe that we need to talk to the old folks and also speak to them immediately before they start to open their stories.

John Ramsey same they asked the police to complete them at their home because Mark Ramsey was ill with sadness in bed "barely being able to walk".

We were prepared to commit suicide and eager to speak with police officers to find the murderer," he told Walters in 2000.

The next thing we had to do at that point, which was to burrow the female children of our offspring. . "JonBenet was laid to rest within Marietta, Georgia, the town of the Ramseys on the 31st of December of 1996.

The next day, her older siblings were on CNN for an interview of associate degree in which they pleaded with the public to help in identifying the murderer of and their daughters.

Patsy Ramsey, the same as they discovered they were the the main suspects in their daughter's murder Patsy Ramsey said she "didn't believe in him".

We tend to be grieving that we are more likely to lose the child we love... and then, for someone who is responsible simply can't believe it could occur," she told CNN in January. 1997.

We were indignant. We are prone to be horrified, added John Ramsey. "How could they have thought this?

We tend to be a family that is traditional. Lou Smit begins to analyze JonBenet's death despite the fact that they deny it that the police continue to believe that the suspects were responsible for JonBenet's murder.

Boulder County The DA of Boulder County Alex Hunter, however, was not convinced and was eager to investigate other theories.

Three months after JonBenet's death was announced, he invited Smit to the fold.

He began to look at the evidence and see possible leads that officers and the public did not have or were not aware of.

It gave the appearance of the fogeys are most likely concerned." Smit same in video diary, he began recording as he investigated the incident.

I thought it was becoming a easy situation. I assumed it would be a slam-dunk and i keep in mind that i should reprove the female children of my offspring.

I am a bit of a joker with her, saying "If someone walked into the house, it's Kriss Kringle who was coming back through the chimney.

However, as Smit began to investigate the incident and began to think that the police should look for a persona non in fact.

He pointed out the unlocked window that was in the basement however , photos showed cobwebs on the windows that would likely have broken if someone was to have slipped through.

The police were not convinced that it was feasible to pass through the window. Smit explained to them that it was due to research the matter himself.

The big problem is whether you were able to use this tiny window - without worrying about this web spider," Garrett aforementioned.

The answer to this question is" maybe "... but the other important factor is how long the icon was used after JonBenet passed away because spiders reproduce webs extremely fast."

The police also found an image of an Hi-Tec entire boot, which was found close to JonBenet's body . There was no one in the family of this brand's shoes also two marks on his back and face as he mentioned were caused by the use of a weapon.

There's no reason why the Ramseys should have to carry an weapon, so the Ramseys do not have weapons," Smit aforementioned at the time.

If it's not a weapon, then what is it? This is the question I always ask.

In his diaries of his videos, Smit detected that whoever wrote the ransom note had the language used in many films.

Particularly, he noticed the resemblances to the snatch-based drama "Ransom" which was the city of Boulder in the year. In this film, the businessman was a "big cat had his son taken.

There's a lot of verbiage that is constant in this note, as well as the note that was composed in the moving-picture show,"Smit mentioned in the tapes.

The note said: "You aren't the sole wealthy person in the world" It also included various lines that resemble the dialogue in the movies "Dirty Harry" and "Speed".

Smit also spoke about the DNA evidence that police discovered beneath JonBenet's fingernails, as well as his underwear in videos logs.

He mentioned that this proof "was not something that was made public for long enough.

Analyzing his DNA revealed that he doesn't have any kinship with anyone in Ramsey's family. Ramsey family.

Following the first formal interrogation of JonBenet's oldersters in 1998's spring, which was four months after his death they took nearly 2 years to sit before the police for a further interrogation.

They returned for another time within the Gregorian calendar month of 1998 but now, investigators have recorded it on video.

There were many months of talks and discussions determine if they could be recorded or not. What the issues could have to be... should they were. Boulder Police were among them," aforementioned inquiring communicator Carol McKinley.

The Ramseys stated, "We don't trust the police. We don't need police officers in our homes. The interrogation ultimately took place in another local department, and investigators from Boulder were compelled to observe from a different building.

Tom Haney, a detective in Tom Haney, a detective with the Mile-High City local department, interrogated the victim Ramsey while Smit John Ramsey was interrogated by Smit John Ramsey.

In each question JonBenet's family members strongly denied that any member of their family had killed their daughter.

When Haney suggested that there could be evidence to could connect Patsy Ramsey to the murder of her daughter Patsy Ramsey responded, "It's totally impossible.

Go retest. He claimed she had told him that it was not possible to provide "physical evidence" connecting her to the crime.

The investigators did not find any evidence of incrimination during the interrogation by the Ramseys.

Smit's daughter Cindy Marra, said the interviews "confirmed her conviction that the Ramseys did not have anything to do" in the murder of JonBenet. "I'm not saying that parents shouldn't murder their children... Parents murder their children," Smit said in his tapes.

The officers are trying prove that Patsy is responsible. ... The actions they took before, during , and following the death of JonBenet are acceptable to innocent people. ... The suspects didn't do it.

While the investigation was ongoing under Smit Marra, he was worried that the authorities had excluded any possibility that an intrusion could have led to murdering Jon Benet, and therefore were not looking for evidence to support the potential, Marra said.

I believed there was something amiss at any point and there was an utter injustice," he said in the recordings. "I saw the evidence of an intrusion inside the home the night before.

The hacker theory he had developed about JonBenet's murder being increasingly thrown aside, Smit ultimately chose to quit the investigation. He wrote in an email addressed to Boulder Hunter District Attorney:

Although I would like to remain involved with the investigation to help locate JonBenet's killer I am of the opinion that I can't with absolute conviction be a one of those who are being targeted by innocent individuals, "said Smit, referring to JonBenet's parents.

"It is completely unsuitable and unmoral for me to remain in the position I am in even if I believe so strongly in it."

However, even as he took a step off of his official position in the matter Marra continued to call for justice for JonBenet and stood at the side of his parents, Marra said.

When Hunter requested an inquiry by a grand jury their evidence back in 1998, almost two years following JonBenet's murder, they were able to listen to the intruder theory of Smit.

However, just like the police, jurors did not believe that anyone would have walked through the window without the cobwebs still in place.

Jonathan Webb, one among the jurors of the grand jury, claimed on "20/20" about Smit's theory of persona non grata made no sense to someone to go through a small window in this way and not touch the webs "would be exceptional," he said.

The jury all over the accusatory John and the chump Ramsey of illegally, recklessly or recklessly allowing the child to be placed in a situation of circumstance that is threatening to the child's health or life" and "to assist anyone with the aim of delaying, preventing or preventing the development or detention, arrest, prosecution, conviction, and punishment of that individual to be punished for the committing of a crime. However, while the jury may believe that the parent who was guilty was guilty and in addition, the alternative could have helped however, they couldn't say the United Nations agency did what it did, and Hunter eventually ruled that they didn't have sufficient evidence to lodge an action against the elderly.

In the following years, Smit continuing to review his knowledge regarding the

JonBenet case , and then compiled the details into a report.

He believed the answer to JonBenet's killer was in the deoxyribonucleic acid that was found in his underclothes and under his fingernails.

A substitute deoxyribonucleic acid testing technique was invented, dubbed tactile deoxyribonucleic acids that enabled consultants in rhetoric to examine dead skin cells found on the objects of crime scene.

Mary Lacy, the Boulder public prosecutor at the time, was set to conduct this check on JonBenet's pajama-leggings. the results were positive for at most one male deoxyribonucleic acid that was not identified likely even two.

It was at the time of this check was made that Lacy sent an open letter in the name of John Ramsey stating that his workplace did not include his spouse, him the chump Ramsey or anyone else from their immediate family members to be suspect of the death of JonBenet.

Patsy Ramsey passed away from the female reproductive organs of her body in 2006. She was buried beside JonBenet in Georgia JonBenet's father John Saint Andrew Ramsey aforementioned.

Lou Smit dies, however the investigation continues. After 13 years. Smit believed it was possible that Associate in nursing, an unidentified persona non grata is responsible for the murder of JonBenet.

But he was also not getting enough time. His diagnosis came from cancer in the year 2010.

But despite the fact that a plethora of people came to pay respect to him at the medical facility, as well later in his hospice care, he had never ever stopped talking about the case of JonBenet as per his alternate male offspring Dawn Miller.

Marra stated that prior to his death, while in his hospital bed, he informed her he needed someone else to work on the case.

He said, "I require someone to investigate this issue. Do not let him pass away, "she said.

He then requested Pine Tree State to jot down a name, and I did. I picked up an eraser and a piece of paper. handed Pine Tree State a reputation and then he said, "Start therewith name."

Smit passed away on Aug. 11 on the 11th of August, 2010.

Marra stated that following her death her family teamed up with Smit's former murderers to investigate the matter.

We all share the desire to see Lou's final wish that this issue never dies with him," said John Anderson an Smit's friend and ex- El Paso County Sheriff in Texas.

It's this dedication to respect, love for Lou that keeps our team going forward.

The team was able to refer to the databases Smit had developed to begin with identifying suspects.

One of the names on the list included Gary Oliva, a homeless man who was a member of the same church for less than two blocks from Ramsey's residence and also told a acquaintance via phone shortly after JonBenet's death "he'd just killed a young girl, McKinley mentioned.

Authorities finally have since cleared Oliva for being a possible suspect, despite not being able to link them to the murder scene.

Bill McReynolds, a man who dressed as Santa at Christmas time during The Ramseys during three consecutive years was also under investigation, but ultimately cleared because his DNA was not in line with the ones found by investigators.

Michael Helgoth, who owned two pairs of Hi-Tec boots as well as a stun gun , and who committed suicide just after JonBenet's murder He was cleared of the crime after investigators discovered that his DNA was not in line with to the DNA found in the area of murder. "We looked through the names of people that were suspects... before we then got to our top 20.

In the present, from the top 20 choices, what our team's focus was on collecting DNA samples and DNA tests." Anderson said. Anderson said.

We are not detectives. We do not question possible suspects.

Any information we come across that has matches will be sent immediately to Boulder district attorney as well as the Boulder Police Department and they will follow it up.

We're trying to remove individuals off the list, and we're thinking that if we go on hoping to reduce it to just one person who is still on this checklist," Marra said.

Anderson stated that the team who identified Smit's suspects had a meeting with police at Boulder in September of 2020 to make a list of the top 20 suspects in this investigation.

Marra claimed that she didn't think "at at this point that they are currently examining the matter".

When asked for comment When asked about their response, officials from the

Boulder Police Department said there is an ongoing and active investigation into the murder of JonBenet; However, the department has never made public statements about the investigation's handling.

Marra is convinced that her daughter, who are Smit's granddaughters are going to fulfill her final wish, even if they're unable to.

My children... can continue to pursue this endeavor until we're too old for this," Marra said. "But we're not planning to stop looking into it.

We're not going to make it happen. After the death of their child, John Ramsey lost his job. He claims having spent millions on lawyers, private investigators and security.

JonBenet's half brother John Andrew Ramsey said his father had been married and was focussed on his living a normal life, he also stated that their struggle for justice for his half-sister had not been over.

The family hasn't lost the determination to fight, and also the determination... for track down the murderer," said John Andrew Ramsey. "We are engaged in daily investigations.

There are a group of committed volunteers who participate on a daily basis.

I believe it's vital to let people know the issue can be solved," he continued.

There's a myth that this is a murder that is not solved and that we should believe it to be true but it's not the reality.

If we make use of the evidence and take a look at the facts, and we'll discover this killer. "

Chapter 8: CONNECTICUT: Mary Badaracco disappeared

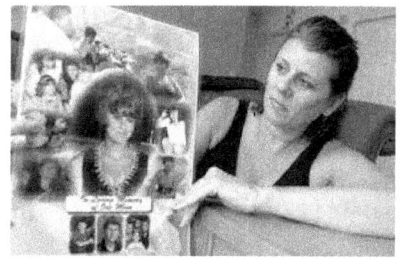

SHERMAN - Prior to Helle Crafts was a victim of the wood chipper in 1986, and before Regina Brown went missing without any trace in 1987, just five months following the time Elizabeth Heath was reported missing by her husband in 1984, there was the mystery in the case of Mary Badaracco.

In the 27 years that have passed since her disappearance, 38-year old Sherman woman Richard Crafts was convicted of murdering his wife. He was sentenced to a minimum of 50 years in prison. In April of 2010, the body of Heath was discovered under a barn at the Newtown estate where she was living.

His murder is currently being investigated. However, Badaracco, just like Brown has not been reported or seen again despite an investigation which may be close to concluding some of the concerns his daughters have dealt for more than three decades.

The week before, The News-Times learned that the one-man grand jury summoned witnesses find the answer to one of the area's most difficult mysteries that remain unsolved. Since the grand jury's sessions are conducted in the dark, neither investigator nor official can verify the legitimacy of the grand jury.

It's one of those moments in your professional life that you will never ever forget." told former State Police Major Peter Warren, who was a road trooper in his early years stationed at Southbury Barracks when the Badaracco's daughters, Sherrie and Beth, are now Sherrie Passaro as well as Beth Profeta visited the barracks during Labor Day weekend in 1986 to inform their mother of her illness. While the circumstances that involve Crafts, Brown, Heath and Badaracco aren't connected however, there are similarities.

The wives were married to couples that were dissolving Three of the husbands three of the husbands - Badaracco, Brown and Heath separated when their wives divorced.

The disappearance of the infamous Badaracco was classified as murder in the year 1990, however, the reward of $20,000 - later increased to $50,000 but not enough to entice anyone who has information about the fate of Badaracco or may lead authorities to the body of his.

The husband of the Badaraccos, Dominic Sr., who was the owner of a bar and house-covering business in Danbury in Connecticut, said to that the Superior Court judge who divorced in May 1985 that he returned to work nine months prior to discover that his wife of 15 years gone.

The home located on Wakeman Hill Road where they were staying for the last one year was lacking more than $ 100,000 in cash as well as other valuables they agreed to before leaving, he told the judge.

The only thing that was left was his car keys as well as the wedding engagement ring.

'LET THEM PROVE IT'

The house located on Wakeman Hill Road wherever that they resided for the last six months was missing more than $ one hundred thousand in cash and various things that they had agreed to prior to his departure and told the judge.

The only thing that was left were his keys to his car and the wedding ring he wore in the years after The Virgin Badaracco went missing The investigation has been sporadic in become publicized.

In the years following her disappearance, she vanished, police from the state conducted an investigation into a former member from the Port chapter of Hells Angels motorbike gang, UN agency informed them that Joseph Badaracco, one amongst Dominic's sons UN agency was an Hells Angel, and another member of the gang "whacked" The Virgin Badaracco on the advice of his father.

If the police believe they killed his stepparents, "Let them prove it," Joseph Badaracco aforesaid in the last week when asked about the prior claim.

He further confirmed that he'd been subpoenaed for testimony before the jury in the last month but was still to do so due because of his condition.

In the last three years the state police have spent more than $35,000 to exhume the backyards of houses that are located within Newtown as well as New Fairfield, supported a suggestion of Ernie Dachenhausen, a Danbury excavation contractor UN agency that often was employed by Saint Dominic Badaracco, had buried The Virgin Badaracco's car that was missing and was believed to have evidence related to her disappearance.

While the car wasn't located during the searches, Dachenhausen was charged with being a suspect in the murder investigation. The case went without proof in Danbury court in 2009.

In the course of the trial, which concluded with Dachenhausen's verdict, Western District Major Crime Squad

Detective Joseph Bukowski -- for the first time is known as Saint Dominic Badaracco since he was the main suspect in his wife's murder.

My primary suspect would be Saint Dominic Badaracco Sr., UN agency is that the person who was last to verify the victim's health, had an alleged history of adulterous relationships and even force" And UN agency did not provide accurate information to the police Bukowski mentioned above.

The repeated efforts of The News-Times to succeed in the case of the chief Badaracco failed and he's repeatedly refused to take the case up.

Joseph Badaracco aforesaid his family is being harassed by Bukowski. "The person is not in control," he said.

A MOTHER VANISHES

Sherrie Passaro as well as letter Profeta never believed that their mother had fled. "Something was not right.

She won't be attempting this." similar Profeta, World Health Organization is currently residing in Torrington.

Profeta was born recently to the mother from Madonna Badaracco, whom she revered in addition, Passaro had recently been engaged. which was an event that her mother was looking forward to with excitement.

Dominic Badaracco, unmarried and father of four and his future spouse later Madonna Smith, conjointly unmarried and mother of two young daughters, in an establishment where he held hands. They got married in 1970.

Although the word wasn't widely used in the early days, Madonna Badaracco was a battered young woman, Profeta same. She endured many years of abuse at the from the brutality of Badaracco. She would sometimes take U.S.A. and we would leave the property, but Dominic constantly found her." Profeta same.

Both daughters lived being worried about their stepfathers. They were also quarantined currently as they got old. "He's consistently been accountable and very dominating," Passaro same.

If we don't perform something then we tend to not do it.

My mommy was constantly trying to protect U.S.A... About six months prior to Madonna's disappearance She along with Dominic relocated to the house located on Wakeman Hill Road that he purchased the year before.

She worked part-time in the improvement of homes for a local land agent and spent a lot hours painting or working in alternative craft projects.

Passaro, World Health Organization may be one an additional year younger than her sibling. initially learning about her mother's disappearance at the time Dominic Badaracco last saw his associate degreed while receiving an unusual call from the Badaracco lady, Donna.

We were both engaged. my sister was known as American state and the same pa wanted to talk to U.S.A. about weddings. My first question was "Why didn't my mommy contact me? '", Passaro same.

It was a bit strange." The following day at she was at work, Passaro visited Sherman's house but there was no one to please her. While she was there she spotted her mother's 1982 Vex Cavalier was placed on the highway and the driver's windscreen was broken.

The next thing that happened is not clear, Passaro same, partially due to the fact that her anger, but it was also due to the events that took place, see you later all by yourself.

Dominic Badaracco has finally arrived. According to what Passaro recalls the conversation, it went something like this: "Your mother is gone.

He requested Passaro to return to his home later, and empty the things belonging to his mother.

But once she had done that the shopping, every item of her personal products was gone. Likewise, the closets and drawers were empty.

The only thing left was Madonna Badaracco's art pieces as well as a few empty perfume bottles. Badaracco shared with Passaro:

Don't share your information with anyone. Do not reveal your sister's name. My professional will be in charge of everything." she recalls.

Insecure and still scared by her dad figure Passaro was silent. Profeta did not know anything about the disappearance until her sister reached out to her.

In the end, fear for their mother's health was enough to calm them and they called the state police.

A Biker is a great help

Following the sisters' filing of the missing persons report, Sherman's soldier in residence and an officer from the state police were at Badaracco's residence in the evening. Dominic Badaracco repeated his runaway wife's tale.

The Gray Horseman was there Badaracco also admitted to hitting the windshield with his fist in anger.

However, since there was no evidence that Mary Badaracco was the victim of a crime The police were unable to take the car away.

In the end, the vehicle disappeared , and its absence together with any evidence it could contain - has hampered investigators until today.

Bukowski stated that he had spent "an amazing amount of period of" trying to find the Cavalier but there was no evidence of the transfer or sale in Department of Motor Vehicles records.

Disappointed by the absence of progress in the probe, Passaro and Profeta contacted the state representative Lynn Taborsak of Danbury, who, in 1990, succeeded in pressuring the police department of Danbury to declare the case as a murder.

Governor William O'Neill even offered a reward of $20,000 for information that leads to the capture of the Badaracco killer.

Taborsak mentioned that his intervention was at a cost.

I was hit with a brick into my window," she said, and one of the children of Dominic Badaracco, United Nations agency, played Industrial League softball with one of Taborsak's sons. claimed.

Her mother is expected to take care of her own affairs.

Taborsak said the incident to the police, but there was no charge ever imposed. Despite the lack of apparent advancement, the police remain actively.

In 1986, the investigators got information from an Hells Angels associate within the federal witness protection program.

The witness was able to tell the police they were told that Joseph Badaracco and another member, Steve biochemist, killed Madonna Badaracco at her husband's bid to allowing police to access information that was compromising about him.

Kendall, United Nations agency was also in jail at the time. He declined to be interviewed, however, he did a polygraph glance at, which he did not succeed in.

The medical instrument examiner mentioned the biochemist's song after he said that he'd never seen Madonna Badaracco and was unsure whether someone from the bike gang killed her.

Profeta mentioned that she acquired this information when an envelope with maintenance reports was discovered in 1993, when she was responding to request for data on documents related to the case.

It was just in the mailbox. But when I finally received the reports I used be looking for, all names were blacked-out," she added.

Kendall died in a horribly bike crash 18 years ago and which was mentioned earlier Joseph Badaracco.

Badaracco stated that neither he nor any of his relatives was in any way responsible as they were also interested in finding out what happened to his mother.

"ONE PHONE CALL AWAY'

Today, Dachenhausen remains the sole person facing criminal charges in the Badaracco case.

In 2003, the state police received an anonymous request from a man who claimed as he heard the contractor talk about the concealment of an auto for Badaracco.

Bukowski who was appointed to take over the case the following August, finally contacted Dachenhausen initially did not respond to the tipper's request but later admitted that he had dug up three or 4 cars in an estate he held closely in Newtown at the time. The Virgin Badaracco is missing.

One of the vehicles was one of the cars was a Blue Cavalier, he said that it had an outline that was close to the vehicle that it was missing to make police look for it.

After a few days of searching out, police uncovered three cars, but none of them was the Cavalier.

Dachenhausen and the police who supplied false information regarding the location of the vehicles located on the property. was never proven guilty in Apr 2009 of obstruction to the investigation.

The verdict of her jury resulted in a natural incident for the investigators who been hoping that a conviction would give the opportunity to obtain more details about The Virgin's death.

Despite their displeasure at the outcome, Profeta and Passaro stay confident that the matter will eventually be settled and their mother will be discovered.

Major Warren Hyatt, commander of the Western District Major Crime Squad The investigation is in progress.

We're always grateful for what people are willing to share with US. In most cases, you're just an email away.

"The Queen of Hearts

Mary Badaracco's picture along with a brief synopsis of her story are included in the form of "cold case" playing cards which were handed out through the State Department of Corrections last year to more than 18,000 prisoners from the state.

The State Prison System. The goal is that playing cards will lead to new leads in the Badaracco case as well as other cases. The Badaracco card is considered to be the Queen in the deck.

The CUE Center for Missing Persons In addition, the CUE Center for Missing Persons has launched an online site, MaryBadaracco.com, which provides details about the case as well as gives people the ability to provide advice anonymously.

Chapter 9: DELAWARE: Jane Marie Prichard

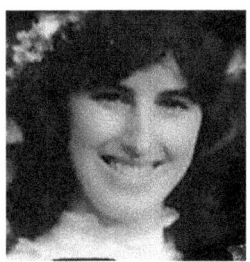

Couple who are from Perth Amboy, New Jersey had planned an autumn trip for habitation in the Delaware Blackbird State Forest a few miles to the south of Middletown and headed heading out on a warm Sat afternoon, with a light breeze.

After choosing a spot to put up their tent The couple decided to walk.

Instead of a peaceful stroll between the trails and trees The couple's discovery caused them to scramble to decide the police.

Just twenty feet away from a pathway and they discovered the partially covered bodies of Jane Prichard who was killed by a blast from a scattergun in the back.

She was 28 years old. earlier. It was 1986. His murder remains unclear.

However, the New Castle County Police Department's newest two-man Cold Case team aims to change the way that it operates.

The first investigation was conducted by Detective Thomas Orzechowski and civilian worker spaceman L. Davis, World Health Organization was dismissed from the police force as a senior sergeant and assigned to handle the case.

An outdoor person

Since childhood, her deceased sister "has always been a member of the outside world," the same Keith Prichard, 59, from Calvert County in southern Maryland.

Their parents, Audrey and Bruno Walter Prichard continue to reside in an similar houses on the same 38-acre farm in the rural region close to Barnesville, MD, wherever she was raised with a passion for horses and the natural world.

Jean Marie was notably on the edge of Keith three years older, but she was also on the verge of his elder twin brother Greg along with his younger sister , who was an alphabetic character.

She was a free-lancer and adventurous as her brother recalls her walking across the country by herself when she was a she was a faculty member was in their beloved Datsun 2000 - still unbroken by her family.

She also utilized her mother's talents in the field of the plants. She was working in Brookside Gardens, a distinguished arboretum located in Montgomery County, Maryland, as she pursued her master's education in biology at The faculty Park field at the University of Maryland.

She resided in the city of Maryland which was a suburban area located in Washington, D.C. Her research, which took the student to Blackbird State Forest many times throughout 3 years of study, were focused on a summer vascular plant, also known as ground bean, also known as pork peanut native plant with edible seeds above and below the ground.

In September nineteen in 1986, she drove an all-white and blue Chevrolet sporting coat accompanied by her analytical instrument and the zero of a colleague's in Lewes heading early morning to go to the forest.

At around 7 a.m. she set off on a road that was to the south from Blackbird State Forest Road and discovered an instrument that ran from the back of the truck about 30 yards deep into the forest.

She was interested in the evolution of the plant leaves turning toward the sun.

She was accumulating the final details she required to complete her thesis. the graduation ceremony is scheduled to take place in the next few months.

The recording of his minute-by-minute information abruptly ended at around 10 a.m.

An arrest, a tip

A man was identified as a police officer on a weekday after Prichard's body was found in the forest. He had seen her when he was looking for squirrels in the forest in that morning when she died. He saw another hunter in close proximity to her, who was describing him as a hunter and using a drawing tool to draw a sketch of the deceased, which was published in the press and printed on leaflets.

A large number of hunters were in the forest at the time However, the police quickly wiped on a shooting accident.

The autopsy found that Prichard was swollen to death from gunshot wounds on his neck and shoulder and neck, his death putting him to the death.

Police conducted interviews with nearly 300 individuals, as well as experts employed by DuPont Co. performed an thorough examination of the scatterguns which struck Prichard However, they did not find any.

The forest area surrounding Prichard's Analysis Station has been delineated and cleared, then monitored for several days. Investigators employed metal detectors, and screened the bottom with screens.

They provided unreleased evidence of their findings to FBI located in Washington. The police questioned the squirrel hunter, a man who was in his 20s. World Health Organization lived close to Newark and was custodian for a nearby business twice and were suspicious of what they being referred to as "some contradictions" in the above mentioned information.

In early October, the police accused him of the crime of degree murder and possessing an deadly weapon while they also charged him with committing a crime. He was under arrest and not being released on bail.

New technology explored

One evidence piece that was discovered - a hair - by police officers who were scouting the scene of the crime has raised hopes because of the latest technological advances. "DNA testing was a new concept in the early days," Orzechowski said. Investigator James Hendricks flew with the small and valuable cargo to California due to the fact that, "in 1986, there was just one DNA lab available at that at the time" Orzechowski said. .

Following a warrant for a search executed at the janitor's house of the squirrel hunter's home, the police were willing to put their money on the California laboratory that could match hairs from the crime scene to.

It was among the first cases to use DNA," Orzechowski said. Researchers, however, discovered no matches.

In August 1987 charges against the single and sole suspect were removed.

Police officers, who at the time were conducting over 300 interrogations during the investigation asked for advice and analyzed all the new suspects that were infiltrated the case, but came up with nothing.

In the years that followed in the months that followed, all leads dwindled or were canceled, and the police that was in charge of the case were forced to focus on other cases and the killing of Jean Marie Prichard was moved to the cold file.

Fresh eyes on the case

In the month of October 2014 New Castle County police captain gap. Elmer M. Setting declared the creation of a brand new death squad for putting to death.

Cold Case Unit Cold Case Unit was created to enhance our vigilance the most sensational and unique cases that are involved in murders at New Castle County, notwithstanding when the crime was committed." This was recently set up. .

A veteran investigator with modern eyes and thus the use of the latest technology is prepared to assist in solving these crimes of a horrific nature and bring an end to the families of the victims," he said.

With a detective on a regular basis and a small number of support staff, the team will be expected to try to locate leads in the most new files or a specific person who could be solved by technological advances that were not available in the moment the crimes were committed. .

The police department of the county includes forty to fifty unsolved murders, beginning in 1971.

In the past they were handled by detectives in addition to their ongoing investigation.

The thought of a special department to focus on unsolved murder cases - defined as those that involve suspicious deaths, that have no suspects with a better reputation and each leads exhausted - been discussed within the local police department for several years prior to when Setting decides to turn it into to become a possibility.

The family members of the victims region is not forgotten." The setting the preceding.

We are able to continue working to bring justice to the perpetrators of these crimes and destroyed countless lives.

Cold case duo

Detective for almost the entire nine-year period, Orzechowski worked as a long-time police officer who worked in the area of major crimes such as active home invasions thefts and rapes - when he was approached regarding the murder unit.

I was truly honored," he said, and he jumped at the chance to accept the job. The cadre is now the most well-known face of the civilian staff position of the unit.

Davis was retired after twenty years in the police force, which included significant detective and crime work.

Also, he had a 20-year run of the family business founded by his grandmother. Four Acres Trailer Sales in Stanton.

He retired in March of 2014 and was joined by his sister, who is now the manager of the company.

When Setting Was conscious of his annoyance about his second attempt to retire set about offering Davis an open position in the case, Davis was overjoyed.

Setting and Davis had a good relationship because of their unique relationship between police and.

"He was my first," Davis said with a smile. "I broke him after he left into the academy.

Davis also stated that "it was an honor " to be asked. The thing that makes the new job thrilling for Davis is the changes in the world.

When I left," he said, "the computers had just come in and DNA testing was available however, it was still at its infancy.

First case of a new unit

The problem that was the main focus of the squirrel hunter's identity in the case of suspects was an the exact issue as the light-emitting diode that led to Prichard's death was considered to be elite due to it was the Cold Case Unit's first investigation was deoxyribonucleic acids.

When Orzechowski and Davis examined what was inside cardboard boxes that were on the shelves of a safe storage space, they both of them believed that the evidence they gathered three decades in the past in the Prichard investigation could have a new possibility.

There's plenty of evidence to suggest that DNA can be produced. DNA." Orzechowski said.

They reached out to family members of the Prichard family. "They were delighted to learn that we didn't abandon the case, and that the investigation is ongoing," Orzechowski said.

After calling, Keith Prichard said: "I thought it was awe-inspiring. I was stunned.

However, Keith Prichard said contact with police was difficult since his sister's murder "certainly left the marks". When they talked about the murder of his father, he said: "It was like it was yesterday.

This conversation brought memories of a memorial plaque in her memory at the botanical gardens where she worked as well as her professor who was finishing her master's thesis. Greg's brother Greg was unconvinced, he added.

After having read about the heartless frauds that target families of victims following the 9/11 attacks, Keith said, Greg was thinking that the call could be fake, coming by someone who was looking to profit from the family in order to gain advantage over the family.

Perhaps from the lingering sadness. Keith is the manager of his father's more than 50 years-old large-format graphics business, is concerned about the pressure of the ongoing investigation into the parents of his, and especially his mother who Keith said was "very emotion-driven ".

He's also concerned about "raising his expectations". But , as Orzechowski and Davis He's curious to know what fresh evidence cutting-edge DNA testing can get from evidence from the past.

A number of articles were sent to unidentified laboratories for testing, Orzechowski said, declining to divulge the specifics.

Davis as well as Davis continued to research the documents, and spoke to Hendricks and others who were involved in the investigation seeking new methods to learn more about what happened.

There haven't been any huge breaks yet, but Davis declared, "You never know.

He said that over time the perpetrator could have spoken to someone about something or someone else who is aware may have divorced a partner whose story was not revealed and has made him more prone to talk about it now.

Setting described the murder of Jane Marie Prichard "tragic" and added: "We hope that the investigation of the evidence gathered in this case will allow us to find and detain the perpetrator of the murder of Jane Marie Prichard..

While Orzechowski And Davis continue to work together Both agree that DNA could offer the answer to solve the murder of Prichard.

It's possible that it will happen quickly. Orzechowski told reporters: "We expect results overnight.

TIPS ARE WANTED

It was reported that the New Castle County Police Department has reissued a sketch of the hunter who was observed with a 28-year-old victim of homicide, Jean Marie Prichard, just before she was killed in the woods within Blackbird State September 20, 1986.

They also showed an article in the News Journal photographs of Prichard and his truck, hoping to gather more information during the cold incident.

Chapter 10: GEORGIA: Vanessa "Honey" Malone

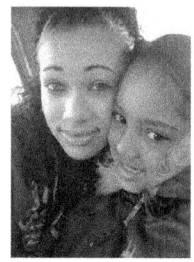

In the case of Vanessa "Honey" Malone's entire family The night of October 23rd, 2012 was just similar to any other night.

Her mother's name is Honey. Flora Malone, picked her daughter aged 18 from her job.

Honey lived alongside her mom living in Stone Mountain, Georgia at that time. They went home to finish their day.

This was until Honey said to her mom that she was planning to go out. Like teenagers, Honey was going out with her friends. She'd done it many nights prior to.

However, this time Honey did not return home. The night began innocently enough: Honey was very tired when she returned home from work . Her mother was puzzled that she was suddenly compelled to go out. today, nobody knows who she was planning to meet or the reason for her.

Honey's mother and sister are convinced that anyone who called or texted her enticed her to an apartment at an area resort.

The police aren't sure the reason she moved into this place or how she got there.

Just after Honey went away, Flora said she heard what she initially thought to be fireworks from the neighboring apartment complex.

My mom's like this," Honey's sister Cassaundra Kennedy shared with Dateline.

"When it occurs to her that she has heard something similar to this, she calls us to confirm that everything is fine.

Flora was referred to as Honey However, Honey did not respond. Initially she was not sure if she could trust that at all. It was not the first time Honey's phone was shut off.

When she first began seeing the emergency vehicle, Honey would refer to them as back. Honey didn't eat.

Mater was in a panic,"Cassaundra told Dateline. It was then that Flora noticed a girl playing outside the door.

She gave it to two males: DeKevin, a former adult male from Honey as well as the friend of hers Chris. "They said to Maine the story of what been happening in Honey," same Flora.

Cassaundra stated: "It was around 11:30 pm. When I received a phone call from my friend and the person was crying in a hysterical manner. Cassaundra inquired with her mother about what was happening, and found out she was the victim of one her parents worst fears. came to fruition. "She informed me that Honey was killed.

When they heard of the incident, Cassaundra rushed to the scene of the crime, the Hampton Apartments, which was just behind Honey and Flora's houses.

When I arrived the police did not give us any details. Mom was present to give the police whatever identifying facts she was able to think up, such as the tattoo she had on her hand. "Cassaundra told me," but police are still unable to identify the person who was killed.

The family claimed that it wasn't until 2:05 a.m. that police were able to officially identify her as Vanessa "Honey" Malone.

DeKalb County Police detectives were given the task of investigating and conducting interviews with relatives and friends.

In the course of the investigation, two of Honey's friends who lived in the same apartment in which Honey was murdered, informed police they were victims of a house invasion.

Police say that the couple claimed that three to six individuals dressed in black, and handing guns smashed through the door to their apartment, they tied them up, and then made them go to the bathroom.

As the men searched the home, the police believe Honey was able to spot the Armed robbery.

She ran away and was shot the first time. The couple who were tied in the bathroom claimed to police that they heard screams and then gunshots. DeKalb County Public data Officer Shiera Joseph Campbell claimed Dateline Honey that she had been shot in the back. She was then transported to a room in the back, and then placed in a very tight closet where she was shot again in the chest.

Honey's family members told police they spotted the intruders' disguise and left.

They claimed they waited for many minutes before they were able to tie and let loose even although it's generally considered to be a robbery which turned unhealthy, however Cassaundra states their family does not believe that.

I don't believe it could have been a crime," she told Dateline. "The only issue that was considered was the life of Honey and her mobile phone..

Cassaundra and her mom believe they were lured into this house. "I think someone called her over there and told my mom that she was tired after she got her from the office," her older sister Honey said to Dateline. "Why would you want to leave your house when you're tired?"

Five years later, Flora and Honey's older sister Cassaundra Kennedy remains waiting for someone to come forward to shed some insight into this crime, which they claim is illogical.

Based on Flora, Honey might be somewhat naive about individuals: "Stone Mountain is not an enormous town but Honey was close to everybody.

Since she was tiny, she was required to do was to aware of people. Regarding her daughter, Flora says "she was truly a sweetheart". She didn't think that something unhealthy could befall one of her daughters.

Honey had a shrewd mouth and would have said another thing," Cassaundra aforesaid, in a speculative discussion about what might have transpired in the evening.

As if someone was communicating verbally "I'm going to shoot you", she'd tell you to shoot me and then.

DeKalb County Police ensure this is typically an open case. They also received information this year about an gun that is involved in the criminal investigation.

The weapon has been delivered for testing by Georgia Bureau of Investigation for testing, but the results are yet to be released for free.

Public information Officer Mythologist states that there are questions regarding the way in which the couple who were betrothed in the living spaces could to do with the murder, but there are no arrests in the investigation.

We have to get to get justice on behalf of Honey," Cassaundra told Dateline. "She was just 18 when she died.

She took all sorts of time to figure out what she had to accomplish and to make sure that they ate away from her.

The family has started an Facebook group 'R.I.P. Honey to get suggestions on how to keep Honey's story alive.

My heart aches for her smiling face, her beautiful eyes, and her voice. I miss fighting with her voice "No You can't wear my shoes..

Flora keeps her daughter in mind every day. "If I could have something, I'd rather to see what might come out from it,"" Flora told Dateline. "She didn't have her initials. Her first automobile, her first home, her infant. They were all taken from him.

Chapter 11: Hawaii: Lisa Au's murder

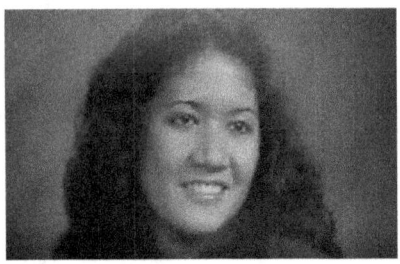

The story is centered about Lisa Au, 19, who was a humble stylist in Kailua, Oahu, and on the evening of January 20 1982 she was about complete her work and was gazing at a torrential downpour rain outside.

After some time, she decided whether to brave the drizzle or not she decided to visit her boyfriend Doug Holmes, who was eating dinner at her sister's home in Makiki.

At midnight, Au and her boyfriend were said to have said goodbye, got in their cars separately and headed for home. But she never made the journey home. And so began the most notorious and unsolved mysteries in Hawaiian history.

When Au did not return home on time the following day, her family contacted Holmes and he informed her that she wasn't home telling her how they said goodbye to the house of her sister and then returned to their homes in their own ways.

The concerned boyfriend then hopped in his car and drove around for hours, driving the roads of the region before he came across Au's car, parked along the highway in Kailua close to a location known as Kapaa Quarry.

Road, however there was no indication of where his girlfriend's location was and authorities were called.

The car's windows were partially opened despite heavy rains that had fallen the night prior, and the interior was inundated with around three inches of water.

In light of the fact that the inside of the vehicle was completely saturated with water, they were shocked to discover that the purse of Au was sitting in the car and was dry, and that he had not his driver's licence and the registration for his vehicle.

Alongside this bizarre discovery, the investigators who examined the vehicle found that it was believed to have be "cleaned" off of fingerprints or other evidence , by somebody.

Because of the suspect nature of the incident, authorities quickly concluded that there was a missing person and possibly a kidnapping and an alert was immediately issued.

In the following 10 days, it would be the largest investigation the state has witnessed, with the police scouring swamps and the wilderness of the area to find all evidence of the woman missing and every day that passed without a ransom request, led the police to be concerned about the most dire.

It was discovered that their fears were established. In January thirty-one 1982 an aspiring runner was running with his dog on Tantalus Drive in Makiki once he stumbled upon the discolored remains of an unadorned body concealed in the brush of Associate in nursing's isolated valley.

Police were able quickly determine the body was Lisa Au, however given the severity of degradation and decay of the body there is no reason why the body was not found. could be determined, regardless of the circumstances. due to the bare condition of her body , and the undisputed fact that she was discovered in a far distance from the vehicle and that it was a certain possibility that it was a case of murder.

The main problem was that nobody had a plan. World Health Organization can be the culprit or even his motives could be once new clues began to appear and theories would start to take flight.

Some of the more interesting of the tips received was from witnesses who stated that in the evening of Au's disappearance they saw his car followed by a second car that was flashing blue lights, reminiscent of police cars.

This interesting detail, when added to the possibility that the window was shut and the purse was empty and the driver's license and registration number were confiscated, led the authorities to believe that the murderer might have been disguised as a police officer , or might have been one of the officers.

The moment this dark theory came to the forefront and spread across the country, there was widespread panic and enormous tension on the department in order to find the culprit.

It was because of the insanity that a mad policeman was snooping around the back roads of the island that the authorities put a lot of effort in attempting to find a police officer who seemed suspicious and was accuse by witnesses that he had harassed women but he never did. no evidence sufficient to warrant an indictment for the incident Au.

Later an individual Au family investigator is said to have found evidence to suggest that the whole pursuit of the officer who was suspect was an act of sabotage, and evidence that there were efforts to lie to the grand jury regarding the sighting of a patrol vehicle or a police officer Au.

It is later revealed that Au was simply oblivious to her driver's licence in the market where she stopped to get home and had not been arrested by a police.

Conclusion

After examining a number of instances during the process of writing this book I believe that one of the most important lessons to be learned is the fact serial killers have existed for many centuries. Maybe it is possible that the Servant Girl Annihilator of 1884 wasn't the first serial killer in the history America. However, it's a good beginning point.

Every chapter of this book has revealed how brutal and calculated serials are in their pursuit to satisfy the craving that which only murders seem to satisfy. It is clear that serial killings aren't only random acts of violence perpetrated by unhinged males. In reality, they are smart enough to be able to conduct their extra-curricular activities in a way that allows them to escape the law.

While I wrote this book I became aware that serial killers although posing a huge threat to the society, are also effective. While this might be seen as uncaring or too clinical, research studies have proven that the increase in serial killers has resulted in rapid change in how police investigation is conducted, moving from simple assumptions to the testing of polygraphs and evidence from forensics.

I hope that regardless of how interesting these stories could be, you've learned something from this book on how serial killers hide themselves. You should always be vigilant about those you have a connection with.

Till next time, stay safe.

www.ingramcontent.com/pod-product-compliance
Lightning Source LLC
Chambersburg PA
CBHW050024130526
44590CB00042B/1889